KETO DIET

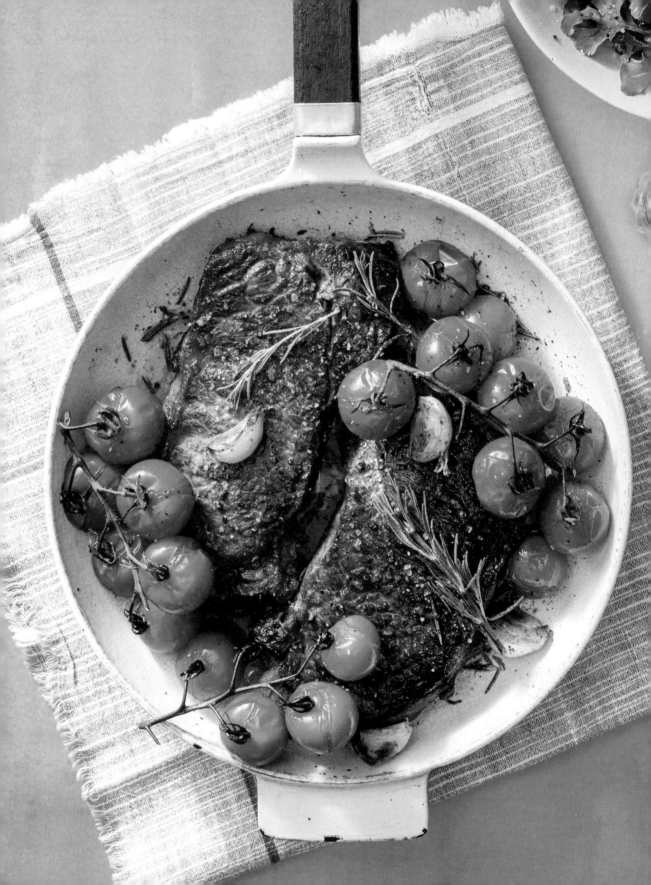

GOOD HOUSEKEEPING

KETO DIET

100+ LOW-CARB, HIGH-FAT RECIPES

★ GOOD FOOD GUARANTEED ★

HEARST
books

HEARSTBOOKS

An Imprint of Sterling Publishing Co., Inc.
1166 Avenue of the Americas
New York, NY 10036

ISBN 978-1-61837-314-4

The Good Housekeeping Cookbook Seal guarantees that the recipes in this publication
meet the strict standards of the Good Housekeeping Institute. The Institute has been a
source of reliable information and a consumer advocate since 1900, and established its seal
of approval in 1909. Every recipe in this publication has been tested until perfect for ease,
reliability, and great taste by the Good Housekeeping Test Kitchen.

Distributed in Canada by Sterling Publishing, Co., Inc.
c/o Canadian Manda Group, 664 Annette Street
Toronto, Ontario M6S 2C8, Canada
Distributed in Australia by NewSouth Books
University of New South Wales, Sydney, NSW 2052, Australia

For information about custom editions, special sales, and premium and corporate
purchases, please contact Sterling Special Sales at 800-805-5489 or
specialsales@sterlingpublishing.com.

Manufactured in China

2 4 6 8 10 9 7 5 3 1

sterlingpublishing.com
goodhousekeeping.com

Cover design by David Ter-Avanesyan
Interior design by Sharon Jacobs

Photography credits: Beatriz Da Costa: 119; Danielle Occhiogrosso Daly: cover, 2, 14, 20,
22, 89, 90, 98, 100, 104; Mike Garten: 6, 10, 28, 32, 38, 42, 52, 58, 60, 64, 68, 70, 72, 76, 78,
86, 96, 106, 108, 112, 116, 124, 127, 130, 133, 137; Getty Images: Iakov Kalinin 44;
© Pernille Loof: 54; © Kate Mathis: 34; © Con Poulos: 80; Emily Kate Roemer: 123;
@ Kate Sears: 134; © Anna Williams: 16

contents

FOREWORD **7**

INTRODUCTION **8**

Breakfast 15

Appetizers & Snacks 33

Poultry 53

Meat 81

Fish 113

Vegetables & Salads 125

INDEX **140**

METRIC CONVERSION CHARTS **143**

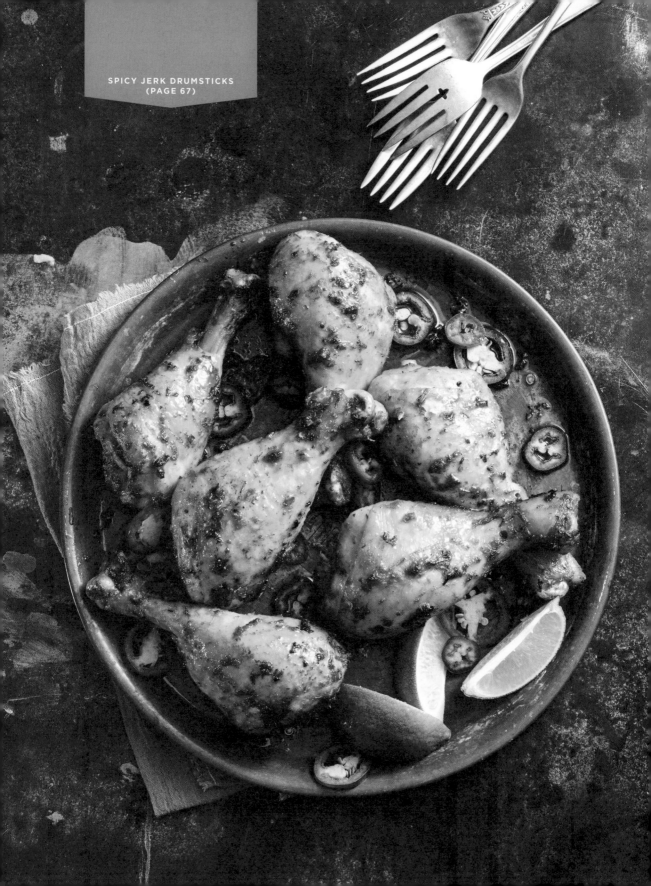

SPICY JERK DRUMSTICKS
(PAGE 67)

Foreword

There's no doubt that the keto diet is having a moment. In fact, as the latest version of carb-restricting gains increasing groundswell, it seems like *everyone* knows someone who's trying it, whether it's Halle Berry or your Uncle Joe. The popular eating plan advises breaking down your daily calories into about 70 percent fats, 20 percent protein, and 10 percent carbs in order to enter a metabolic state called *ketosis*, where your body burns fat for energy instead of its preferred fuel, carbohydrates.

Since using our bodies' own fat stores for energy sounds downright fantastic to most of us, we wanted to know more. Our nutrition lab's deep-dive into the research on keto diets served as our main resource. Turns out, our bodies naturally burn carbs (aka, glucose) for energy, so cutting them radically means we'll need to use a different energy source to keep our organs functioning. When we break down muscle glycogen—the first biochemical reaction of any low-carb diet, we immediately lose water weight. You've heard those touts for so many diets: "Lose 5 pounds your first week!" Well, since our bodies store about 3 grams of water for every gram of glycogen, this explains those first week miracles.

What about extending this diet long-term? Well, weight loss is highly personal and unique to every single one of us, so keto diets may not be for everyone. Of course, we always encourage you to consult with your doctor before starting any weight-loss regime, but if you're currently taking medications for diabetes management, it is absolutely essential that you talk to your endocrinologist before beginning the keto diet. Some medications actually require eating some carbohydrates to ensure your safety.

We know there are many success stories on the keto diet. Celebrities, athletes, and at least one person you know have had success with it. We encourage you to approach weight loss first by considering your lifestyle and shifting toward healthier eating habits through behavioral changes that promote physical, mental, and psychological well-being for life.

That said, the delicious and filling recipes on the following pages will provide you with plenty of inspiration that can help get you on your way to your keto plan *and* help to spark ideas for making changes to your weekly recipes—no matter where you are in your personal health and weight loss journey.

—The editors of *Good Housekeeping*

Introduction

The keto or ketogenic diet has set the health and dieting world ablaze. If you've picked up this book you probably know a bit about the diet. Let's clear up a few basic questions.

WHAT IS THE KETO DIET?

It is a very high-fat, very low-carb, and moderate protein diet that will put your body in a state of ketosis. Some say that it has been in place for millennia—earliest man ate mostly fats and proteins. When comparing it to other plans, many keto dieters say they have achieved greater weight loss, feel full longer, have improved energy, and have fewer cravings. Keto diets vary in specific nutrient breakdown, but most of the calories you'll eat per day will come from dietary fat sources—about 70 percent of your total daily intake. There's a fair amount of data to support the use of the keto diet to aid in the management of pediatric seizure disorders, and some early research that suggests there may be a benefit to some at risk for type 2 diabetes.

WHAT IS KETOSIS?

When your body is using fat as its main source of energy, your body enters a state called ketosis. When you are limiting your carbohydrate intake to around 10 percent, this metabolic state is initiated.

HOW DOES THIS HAPPEN?

When fat is digested and broken down in the body it produces useable energy called ketone bodies, or ketones. This fat can come directly from the food you eat, or from the breakdown of your fat stores.

Typically carbohydrates are converted to glucose and are used as fuel to run the body. Once glucose supplies are depleted—about two to three days into the keto diet—your body will begin using ketones for fuel instead.

The breakdown of fat into energy is similar to the process that dietary carbohydrates undergo when producing glucose to keep your vital organs up and running. So if we're doing a math equation: ketones are to fat what glucose is to carbohydrates. Clinically ketosis is defined as having blood ketone levels above 0.5 mmol/L.

When you're on a ketogenic diet, your body becomes efficient at burning fat for energy. Since fat contains more than double the calories per gram of carbs or protein (9 calories/1 gram of fat compared to 4 calories/1 gram of carb or protein), you will need to eat far less to feel full. Keto diets may also impact your body's hunger hormones, which can make you feel less inclined to graze while you're on the plan. Additionally, since your body readily burns the fat it has stored (the fat you might be trying to shed), it may help with weight-loss efforts. Prioritizing fat for energy may help you maintain stable blood sugar levels, avoiding the energy highs and lows that can occur when eating refined carbs.

WHAT ARE SOME OF THE CHALLENGES?

The water and electrolyte loss your body will experience on this diet can raise your risk of dehydration, which brings on the "keto flu" that most people experience when first starting the diet. You may feel muscle soreness, headache, and constipation, and become moody, lethargic, and have difficulty focusing. You will need to take dietary supplements for the vitamins and minerals you aren't getting from fruit, starchy veggies, and grains, which could raise your risk of disease and bone loss. Note that if and when you go off the diet the hormone shifts you experienced that suppress appetite will be reversed—meaning that you may be hungrier than you were before you started (and thus reverse your weight loss). The keto diet is not for everyone, and we strongly recommend that you consult your physician before starting this plan, especially if you have been diagnosed with type 2 diabetes or rely on exogenous insulin and/or certain types of oral hypoglycemics for disease management.

WHAT ARE RATIOS?

Keto is based on ratios of macronutrients, a.k.a. protein, carbs, and fat. Each provides energy (calories) per gram consumed. Keto dieters aim to receive at least 70 percent of their calories from fat. About 20 percent should come from protein, and the remaining 10 percent from carbs. The number of calories you should eat depends on a few factors, including:

- Lean body mass
- Physical activity and activities of daily living
- The thermic effect of food or the energy your body requires to digest and absorb the food you eat

Many ketogenic-based macro calculators are available online, like tasteaholics.com/keto-calculator and ketogains.com/ketogains-calculator. You can plug your desired outcome (e.g., weight loss or weight maintenance) and get estimates for your calorie needs. Tracking

may help with accountability and can aid in your progress, since it provides a visual record of what you're consuming each day.

SO HOW DO I START EATING KETO?

When planning your daily meals, think eggs or protein-enriched smoothies for breakfast, frittatas or salads for lunch, and fish, steak, or chicken (often with a yummy sauce) with greens or other low-carb vegetables for dinner. But what about dessert? Berries and dairy-rich options are always good picks. When you need a snack or to get your keto ratios up, pop one of our fat bombs (starting on page 46). Grains, starchy veggies, and sweeter fruits are off-limits.

WHAT CAN I DRINK ON THE KETO DIET?

It's crucial to drink plenty of water when beginning the keto diet. You may even notice that you're visiting the bathroom more often, and that's normal! This is linked to depletion of muscle-glycogen stores (your body breaks down glycogen for energy before you tap into fat stores). Since we store about 3 kilograms of water weight per 1 kilogram of muscle, you'll release water into your bloodstream and ultimately eliminate fluid and electrolytes via urine. This excretion can trigger flu-like symptoms, including fatigue, headaches, coughing, sniffles, irritability and/or nausea, and hence it's earned the moniker "keto flu." (Not to worry, these symptoms are unrelated to the influenza virus!) The "keto flu" usually lasts a few days while your metabolism adjusts to prioritize fat for carbs for energy. Beat the symptoms by hydrating and consuming salty foods and electrolytes consistently. →

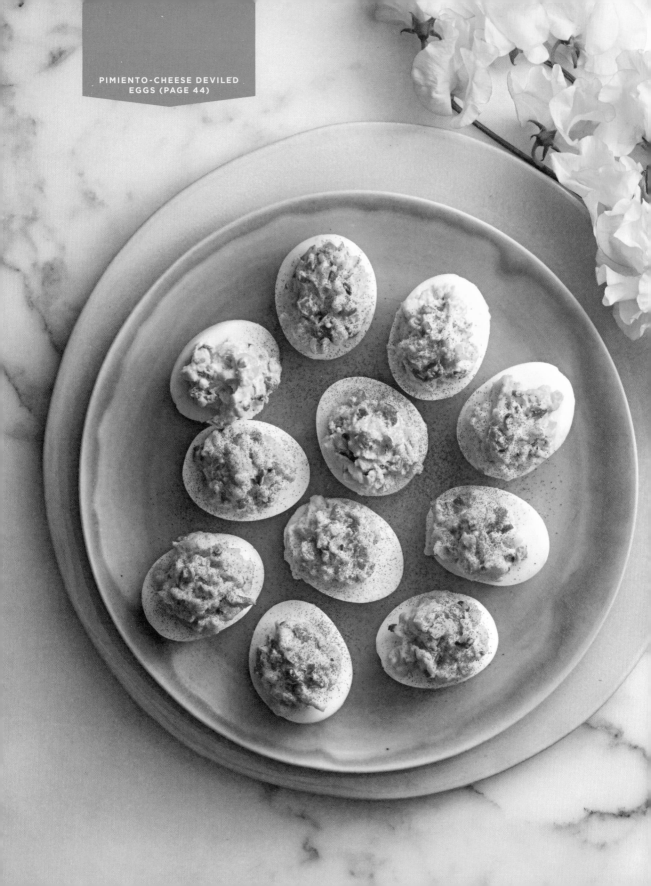

PIMIENTO-CHEESE DEVILED
EGGS (PAGE 44)

Besides water, it is advised to avoid sugary drinks. For coffee and tea, switch to heavy cream or half-and-half to help ease your ratios. Wine and low-carb beer have 3 grams of carbs per serving, so you're often better off with pure spirits like vodka, gin, and tequila, which have zero carbs. Be wary of mixers. As always, drink moderately.

WHEN IS MY BODY IN KETOSIS?

It's important to know if and when you're in ketosis when you first start eating low-carb. Not only is it a great confidence booster, but testing also lets you know whether you're doing things right or wrong and whether you need to make any changes.

An easy test is to sniff for "keto breath." After a few days, you might notice a taste that's somewhat fruity and a bit sour or even metallic. The reason? When your body is in ketosis, it creates the ketone bodies: acetone, acetoacetate, and beta-hydroxybutyrate. Acetone in particular is excreted through your urine and your breath, the latter of which causes "keto breath." The change in the smell of your breath and the taste in your mouth usually diminish after a few weeks.

A more accurate way to determine if you are in ketosis is by using ketone urine test strips. They're fairly inexpensive, and they let you instantly check the ketone levels in your urine. You can find them online or at most pharmacies. Try to take the test a few hours after you wake up in the morning and after you have rehydrated. Being dehydrated after a night's sleep can cause a false positive.

The most accurate test involves a blood ketone meter. This type of test is a bit more of an investment but it's much more accurate, because it tests your blood directly. For nutritional ketosis, your reading should be between 0.5 and 5.0 millimeters.

It's not necessary to check your ketone levels continuously in the long term. Within a few weeks, you'll know if you're eating right and it will become very easy to stay in ketosis.

ANYTHING ELSE I NEED TO KNOW?

As you begin to lose some weight, think about what you can do to feel even healthier. Whatever you're doing now, try to do a little more. Ultimately, whatever activity you choose to do, it's important to stay hydrated—especially on the keto diet—so consider upping your fluid intake by at least two to four cups of H_2O (and electrolytes as needed) for every 30 minutes to an hour of physical activity you do.

If you already exercise, increase the amount and/or intensity of what you do. If you don't exercise at all, start by walking or slow jogging, or a combination of both, for 15 to 20 minutes every other day.

If you already go to the gym or lift weights, add an extra exercise or do some cardio. Try something new, maybe a class or doing an activity like dancing, or playing a sport.

Consistent physical activity will help reduce blood pressure and cholesterol levels as well as reduce risk for various heart diseases and type 2 diabetes—and stress! And your energy level will increase.

The main goal of the keto diet is to keep you in ketosis consistently. For those just starting out, achieving metabolic ketosis may take up to eight weeks.

How to Prepare Your Keto Kitchen

STEP 1:
REMOVE CARB CUES

Give away or toss high-carb foods from your fridge, freezer, and pantry. This includes:

- **Starchy veggies and grains** such as all cereal, pasta, rice, potatoes, corn, oats, quinoa, flour, bread, bagels, wraps, rolls, croissants, and crackers.

- **Legumes like lentils and peas**, beans, and chickpeas.

- **Sugary foods and drinks** such as sugary sodas, sweetened energy drinks, fruit juices, milk and sweetened yogurt, desserts, pastries, milk chocolate, candy bars, etc.

- **Processed fats and oils** such as salad dressings, dips, and premade toppings may contain carbs, so toss them in favor of keto-friendly avocado and coconut oils.

- **High-carb fruits** such as bananas, dates, grapes, mangos, papayas, and all dried fruits like raisins, cranberries, and cherries.

> **TIP**
>
> Sugar alcohols can be easily spotted on a food label as ingredients ending in "—ol."

STEP 2:
SHOP FOR KETO-FRIENDLY WHOLE FOODS

Be sure to read labels! Look at the nutritional information provided on packages to see carb content, sugars, and additives. Stock your fridge and pantry with the following:

- **Beverages** such as water, coffee, and teas.

- **Broths** such as chicken, beef, and bone.

- **Spices and herbs:** Make sure your favorite dried spices and herbs are still fragrant and use fresh when you can.

- **Sweeteners** such as stevia and erythritol.

- **Low-carb condiments** such as mayonnaise, mustard, pesto, and sriracha.

- **Pickled and fermented foods** such as pickles, kimchi, and sauerkraut.

- **Nuts and seeds** such as macadamia nuts, pecans, almonds, walnuts, hazelnuts, pine nuts, flaxseeds, chia seeds, and pumpkin seeds.

- **Meat and poultry** such as chicken, beef, lamb, pork, turkey, and game.

- **Seafood** such as oily fish like salmon and mackerel and shellfish.

- **Eggs**

- **Non-starchy veggies** such as asparagus, broccoli, Brussels sprouts, cauliflower, cucumbers, eggplant, garlic, lettuce, mushrooms, olives, onions, peppers, tomatoes, and zucchini.

- **Low-carb fruits** such as strawberries, raspberries, blackberries, and blueberries. Lemons and limes are good to have on hand for adding flavor to drinks and dishes. Avocados are also lower in net carbs and full of healthy fat.

- **Full-fat dairy** such as butter, sour cream, heavy (whipping) cream, cheese, cream cheese, and unsweetened yogurt and unsweetened plant-based alternatives such as coconut milk.

- **Fats and oils:** Avocado oil, olive oil, butter, coconut oil, ghee, lard, and bacon fat are all great for cooking.

STEP 3:
EQUIP YOUR KITCHEN

Aside from kitchen basics like skillets, pots, and pans here are items that will make keto meal prep faster and easier:

- **Sharp knives:** Most prep time is chopping or slicing. With a sharp chefs' knife, paring knife, and serrated knife, you'll breeze safely through any prep.

- **Food scale:** It will measure solids or liquids and get the perfect amount every time. If you use it in tandem with an app like MyFitnessPal you'll have all the data you need to hit your goals.

- **Food processor:** It is ideal for chopping cauliflower for rice, and pureeing sauces and dressings.

- **Blender:** The tool for morning smoothies, soups, and shakes.

- **Spiralizer:** Make vegetables into noodles or ribbons in seconds.

STEP 4:
PLOT YOUR MEALS FOR EACH DAY

Planning and measuring will impact your success. If you have the ingredients shopped and know what you're making, you're less likely to stray, give up, or order take-out. Plus, you can dream about that cheesecake bomb you'll have for dessert!

After you plan for a few weeks, your body will adjust to how much and what types of food you're eating. After a while you'll find a pattern of what works, what meals you want to repeat, and you'll instinctively know what to eat to stay on track.

To start a keto plan for weight loss and breakdown your macronutrient intake accurately, you can use an online keto calculator (our recommendations are on page 9) before you start, and adjust your meal plan from there. Simply adjust serving sizes to add more or less based on your personal nutrient needs. Or if it's a matter of 100 calories, you can add or subtract a tablespoon of oil or butter when cooking.

> **TIP**
>
> When counting macros, your net carbs are more important to track than total carbs. Net carbs account for the fiber in your food. To calculate, subtract the grams of fiber from the total carbs.

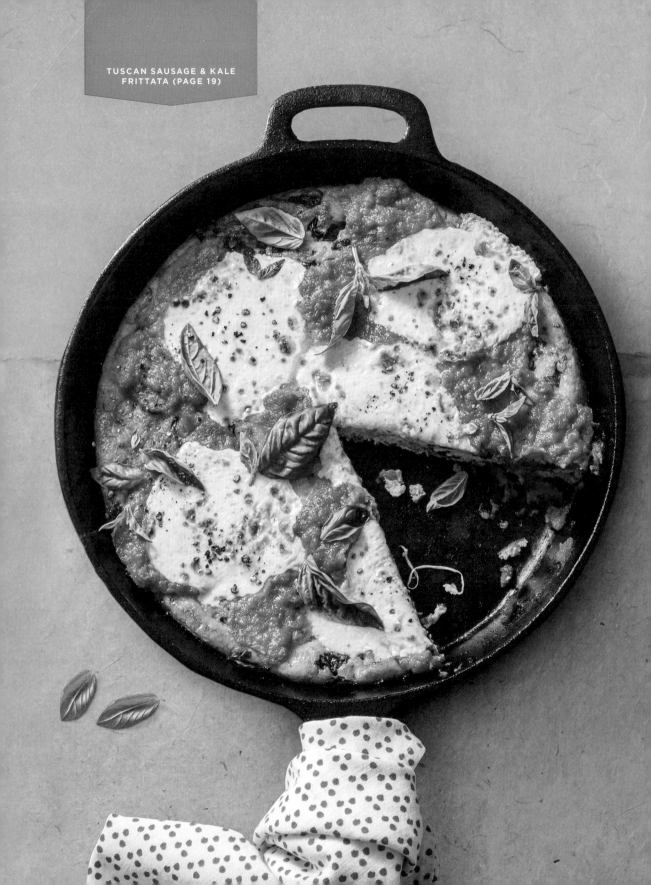

TUSCAN SAUSAGE & KALE
FRITTATA (PAGE 19)

1 | Breakfast

The keto diet, like most diet plans starts with a healthy breakfast. Need breakfast-on-the-run? Grab a couple of our Spinach & Prosciutto Frittata Muffins, yummy at any temperature. Or whip-up a smoothie: Green Light Juice gives you a savory start with its blend of avocado and spinach with a coconut-lime base. If you're in the mood for a fruity sip, Berry Blast Smoothie is your jam. And for those days when dessert for breakfast is calling you—Lemon Cheesecake Smoothie!

When you have more time, gather the family and make Scrambled Eggs with Cream Cheese, Crustless Quiche Lorraine, one of our frittatas, or set up your own omelet bar. A good start will have you ready for keto all day.

Lox Scrambled Eggs 17

Scrambled Eggs with
Cream Cheese 18

Tuscan Sausage & Kale Frittata 19

Summer Squash Frittata 21

Spinach & Prosciutto Frittata
Muffins 23

Basic Omelets 24

Huevos Rancheros 26

Chive & Goat Cheese Frittata 27

Crustless Quiche Lorraine 29

Berry Blast Smoothie 30

Lemon Cheesecake Smoothie 31

Green Light Juice 31

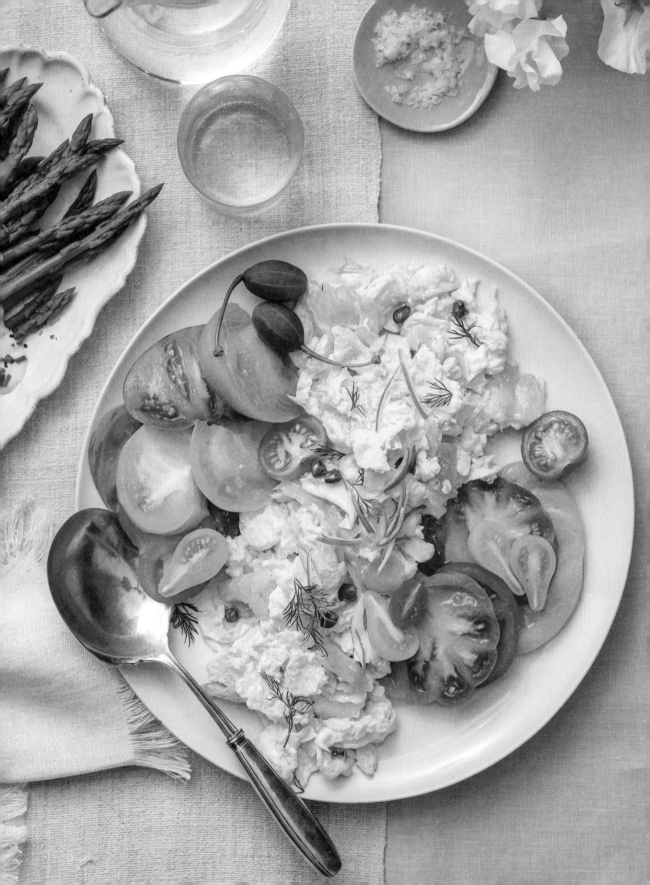

Lox Scrambled Eggs

Move over bagels! Pile this salmon and cream cheese eggstravaganza onto tomato slices and top with your favorite garnishes.

PREP: 20 MINUTES   TOTAL: 25 MINUTES

12 large eggs

2 tablespoons heavy cream

¼ teaspoon kosher salt

1½ tablespoons butter

3 tablespoons cream cheese, crumbled

4 ounces sliced smoked salmon, chopped into small pieces

2 tablespoons finely chopped red onion

1 tablespoon capers, rinsed and chopped

1 tablespoon fresh dill, chopped

2 pounds assorted tomatoes, sliced

1. In a large bowl and using a fork, beat the eggs, cream, and salt until well blended.

2. In a 12-inch nonstick skillet, melt the butter on medium. Add the egg mixture to the skillet and cook, stirring continuously with a spatula, until the eggs are almost cooked, 6 to 8 minutes. Fold in the cream cheese and salmon. Cook 1 minute longer, or until the egg mixture is set but still moist, stirring continuously.

3. Place the eggs on serving platter. Sprinkle the chopped red onion, capers, and dill over the eggs. Garnish with tomatoes.

SERVES 6: About 200 calories, 16g protein, 2g carbohydrates, 16g total fat (7g saturated), 1g fiber, 181mg sodium.

TIP

To round out brunch, serve with steamed or roasted asparagus with Ranch Dressing, page 139.

Scrambled Eggs with Cream Cheese

This is a keto-perfect brunch entrée. Want to make it just for you? Use 2 eggs, 2 teaspoons butter, and 2 tablespoons (1 ounce) cream cheese. Season lightly with salt and pepper.

PREP: 10 MINUTES   TOTAL: 20 MINUTES

14 large eggs

¼ teaspoon ground black pepper

3 tablespoons butter

2 packages (3 ounces each) cream cheese, cut into 1-inch cubes

1. In a large bowl and using a wire whisk, beat the eggs and pepper until well blended.

2. In a 12-inch nonstick skillet, melt the butter on medium; add the eggs. With a heat-safe spatula, gently stir the egg mixture as it begins to set to form soft curds.

3. When the eggs are partially cooked, top with the cream cheese. Continue cooking, stirring occasionally, until the eggs have thickened and no visible liquid egg remains. Serve on a warm platter.

SERVES 8: About 245 calories, 13g protein, 2g carbohydrates, 20g fat (10g saturated), 0g fiber, 217mg sodium.

FUN FLAVORS

Scrambled Eggs with Cream Cheese & Salmon

Prepare as directed above, but sprinkle **4 ounces smoked salmon**, chopped, over the eggs with the cream cheese. To serve, top with ¼ **cup chopped green onions**.

SERVES 8: About 255 calories, 15g protein, 2g carbohydrates, 21g fat (10g saturated), 0g fiber, 321mg sodium.

Tuscan Sausage & Kale Frittata

Pizza goes keto in this yummy egg "pie." Swap in hot sausage if you want to add a little spice to your day. Wrap leftovers in wedges and refrigerate up to 3 days. Microwave for a minute to warm. See photo on page 14.

PREP: 20 MINUTES   TOTAL: 40 MINUTES

12 large eggs

½ cup whole milk

2 ounces Pecorino cheese, grated (about ½ cup)

¼ teaspoon kosher salt

½ teaspoon ground black pepper

2 tablespoons olive oil

1 small onion, finely chopped

½ pound Italian sausage, casings removed

½ large bunch kale, stems discarded and leaves chopped (about 3 cups)

1 cup no-sugar-added marinara sauce

6 ounces fresh mozzarella, sliced

Fresh basil leaves, for garnish

1. Preheat the oven to 350°F.

2. In a large bowl, whisk together the eggs, milk, Pecorino, salt, and pepper.

3. In a large oven-safe skillet (preferably cast-iron), heat the oil on medium. Add the onion, cover, and cook, stirring occasionally, until tender, 5 minutes. Add the sausage and cook, breaking it up with spoon, until browned, about 5 minutes. Add the kale and cook, stirring occasionally, until just wilted, about 1 minute.

4. Reduce the heat to low and add the egg mixture, stirring to distribute the sausage and vegetables. Transfer to the oven and bake until almost set, 18 to 20 minutes. Remove from oven and preheat the broiler.

5. Gently spread the marinara sauce over the frittata, then top with mozzarella. Broil until the cheese is browned and bubbling, 5 minutes. Top with basil and serve immediately.

SERVES 6: About 480 calories, 28g protein, 8g carbohydrates, 37g fat (14g saturated), 2g fiber, 835mg sodium.

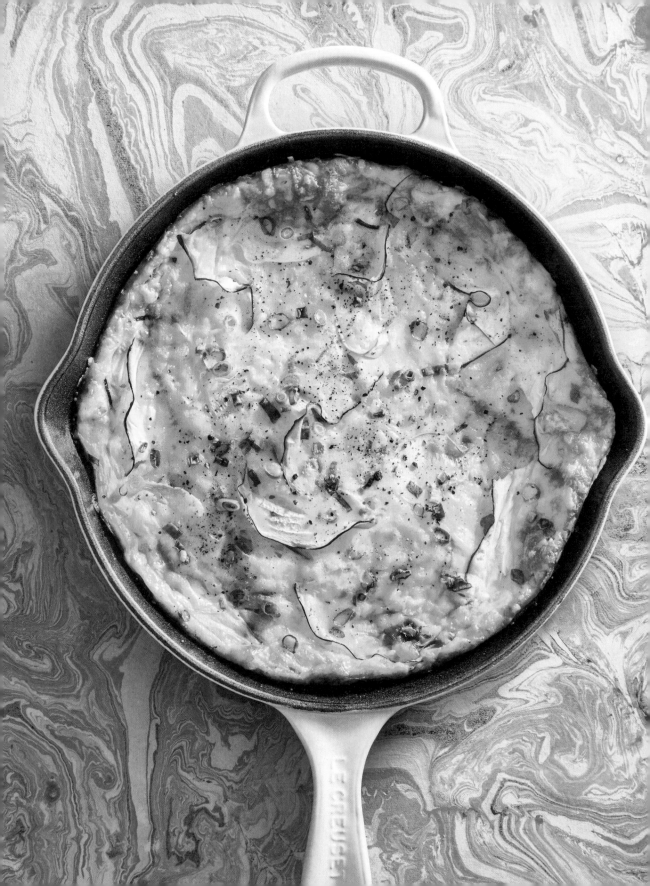

Summer Squash Frittata

Use a combo of zucchini and yellow squash for a visual feast. You can swap in an equal amount of another cheese for the Gruyère if you like.

1½ pounds summer squash,
  very thinly sliced

Kosher salt

8 large eggs

4 ounces Gruyère cheese, shredded

¾ cup whole milk

2 green onions, thinly sliced

¼ teaspoon ground black pepper

1. Preheat the oven to 375°F. In a bowl, toss the squash with ½ teaspoon salt; let stand 10 minutes, then gently squeeze very dry.

2. In a bowl, whisk together the eggs, cheese, milk, green onions, pepper, and ¼ teaspoon salt.

3. Heat a 10-inch oven-safe nonstick skillet on medium. Add the egg mixture. Stir in squash. Cook, occasionally stirring and pulling back the edges, 2 minutes, or until the bottom begins to set. Cook, without stirring, 3 more minutes.

4. Transfer the skillet to the preheated oven; bake 20 to 25 minutes, or until set.

SERVES 8: About 320 calories, 25g protein, 9g carbohydrates, 21g fat (10g saturated), 2g fiber, 690mg sodium.

TIP

Use a mandoline to thinly slice the summer squash.

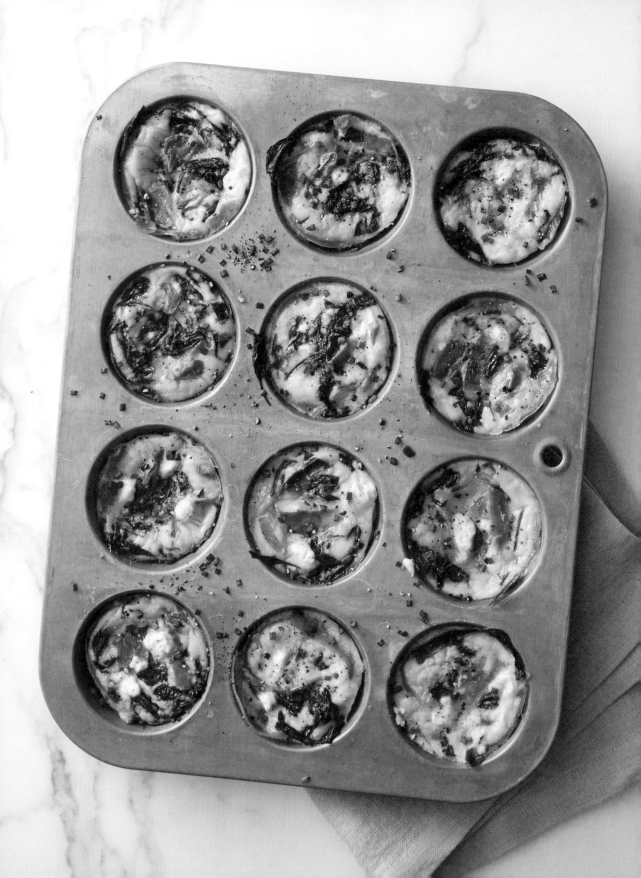

Spinach & Prosciutto Frittata Muffins

These tasty bake-and-take egg cups are packed with protein.
Make a batch on Sunday, then heat and eat them all week.

PREP: **20 MINUTES**   TOTAL: **50 MINUTES**

Nonstick cooking spray

6 large eggs

½ cup whole milk

¼ teaspoon kosher salt

⅛ teaspoon ground black pepper

¾ cup soft goat cheese, crumbled

5 ounces baby spinach, wilted and chopped

½ cup roasted red pepper, diced

2 ounces prosciutto, sliced into ribbons

1. Preheat the oven to 350°F. Spray a 12-cup muffin pan with nonstick cooking spray.

2. In large bowl, beat the eggs, milk, salt, and black pepper. Stir in the cheese, spinach, and roasted red pepper.

3. Divide the batter evenly among the muffin cups (about ¼ cup each), top with some prosciutto, and bake 20 to 25 minutes, or until just set in the center.

4. Cool on a wire rack 5 minutes, then remove them from the cups. Serve warm. These can be refrigerated up to 4 days; to reheat, microwave on High 30 seconds.

SERVES 6: About 155 calories, 13g protein, 4g carbohydrates, 10g fat (4g saturated), 1g fiber, 520mg sodium.

Basic Omelets

Omelets are a perfect keto canvas. Choose a low-carb filling or create your own.

Choice of filling (see options at right)

8 large eggs

½ cup water

½ teaspoon kosher salt

4 teaspoons butter

1. Prepare the filling of your choice; keep warm. In a medium bowl and using a wire whisk, beat the eggs, water, and salt.

2. In a 10-inch nonstick skillet, melt 1 teaspoon butter over medium-high heat. Pour ½ cup of the egg mixture into the skillet for each omelet. Cook, gently lifting the edge of the eggs with a heat-safe rubber spatula and tilting the pan to allow the uncooked eggs to run underneath, until the eggs are set, about 1 minute. Spoon one-fourth of the filling over half the omelet. Fold the unfilled half of the omelet over the filling and slide it onto a warm plate. Repeat with the remaining butter, egg mixture, and filling. If desired, keep the finished omelets warm in a preheated 200°F oven until all omelets are cooked.

SERVES 4 (without filling): About 185 calories, 13g protein, 1g carbohydrates, 14g fat (5g saturated), 0g fiber, 455mg sodium.

FUN FILLINGS

Creamy Mushroom Filling

In a 10-inch nonstick skillet, melt **1 tablespoon butter** over medium heat. Add **1 medium onion**, finely chopped; cook until tender, about 5 minutes. Stir in **8 ounces mushrooms**, trimmed and thinly sliced; **¼ teaspoon kosher salt**; and **⅛ teaspoon ground black pepper**; cook until the liquid has evaporated. Stir in **¼ cup heavy cream**; boil until thickened, about 3 minutes. Stir in **2 tablespoons chopped fresh parsley**. Use one-fourth of the mushroom mixture for each omelet.

SERVES 4: About 290 calories, 15g protein, 8g carbohydrates, 23g fat (11g saturated), 1g fiber, 637mg sodium.

Salsa-Avocado Filling

In a 10-inch nonstick skillet, cook **1 cup medium-hot no-sugar-added salsa** over medium heat, stirring frequently until the liquid has evaporated. Divide the salsa, **1 ripe medium avocado**, peeled and chopped, and **¼ cup sour cream** among the omelets.

SERVES 4: About 300 calories, 14g protein, 10g carbohydrates, 23g fat (8g saturated), 3g fiber, 620mg sodium.

Red Pepper & Goat Cheese Filling

In a 10-inch nonstick skillet, melt **2 teaspoons butter** over medium heat. Add **2 red bell peppers**, thinly sliced, and **¼ teaspoon kosher salt**; cook until tender and lightly browned. Add **1 clove garlic**, finely chopped; cook 1 minute. Divide the red pepper; **2 ounces goat cheese**, crumbled; and **½ cup loosely packed, trimmed, and torn arugula** among the omelets.

SERVES 4: About 260 calories, 16g protein, 3g carbohydrates, 20g fat (10g saturated), 1g fiber, 692mg sodium.

Garden-Vegetable Filling

In a 10-inch nonstick skillet, heat **1 tablespoon olive oil** over medium heat. Add **1 small onion**, chopped; **1 small zucchini**, chopped; **1 small yellow bell pepper**, chopped; **⅛ teaspoon kosher salt**; and **⅛ teaspoon ground black pepper**. Cook until the vegetables are tender, about 10 minutes. Stir in **2 ripe plum tomatoes**, chopped, and **¼ cup chopped fresh basil**; heat through. Use one-fourth of the mixture for each omelet.

SERVES 4: About 240 calories, 14g protein, 7g carbohydrates, 17g fat (6g saturated), 2g fiber, 749mg sodium.

Western Filling

In a 10-inch nonstick skillet, heat **1 tablespoon olive oil** over medium heat. Add **1 small onion**, chopped; **1 green bell pepper**, chopped; **8 ounces mushrooms**, trimmed and thinly sliced; and **¼ teaspoon kosher salt**. Cook until the vegetables are tender and the liquid has evaporated, about 10 minutes. Add **4 ounces sliced ham**, finely chopped (1 cup); heat through. Use one-fourth of the mixture for each omelet.

SERVES 4: About 300 calories, 14g protein, 10g carbohydrates, 23g fat (8g saturated), 3g fiber, 620mg sodium.

INGREDIENT IDEAS

QUICK NO-COOK FILLINGS FOR OMELETS

Here are delicious flavor combos to suit every taste.

- Chopped tomato, crumbled feta cheese, and dill

- Chopped smoked turkey, thinly sliced red onion, and cubed Brie cheese

- Diced ham, chopped green onions, and shredded pepper Jack cheese

- Ricotta cheese and berries

- Chopped fresh herbs, green onions, and sour cream

- Chopped tomato and pesto

- Chopped smoked salmon, cubed cream cheese, and capers

Huevos Rancheros

Avocados are rich in healthy monounsaturated fats and packed with antioxidants. If you're looking to up your ratios, increase to half an avocado per person. You'll add 60 calories, another 5 grams of fat, and 5 of fiber.

PREP: 10 MINUTES   TOTAL: 30 MINUTES

1 tablespoon vegetable oil

1 medium onion, coarsely chopped

1 clove garlic, finely chopped

1 jalapeño chili, seeded and finely chopped

1 can (14 to 16 ounces) tomatoes

¼ teaspoon kosher salt

3 tablespoons butter

4 large eggs

2 tablespoons sour cream

1 tablespoon chopped fresh cilantro

1 ripe medium avocado, pitted, peeled, and cut crosswise into thin slices, for garnish

1. Preheat the oven to 350°F. In a 2-quart nonreactive saucepan, heat the oil on medium-high. Add the onion, garlic, and jalapeño and cook, stirring occasionally, until the onion is tender, about 5 minutes. Stir in the tomatoes with their juices and the salt; heat to boiling over high heat, breaking up the tomatoes with the side of a spoon. Reduce the heat; cover and simmer, stirring occasionally, for 5 minutes.

2. Meanwhile, in a 10-inch skillet, melt the butter over medium heat. Break 1 egg into a small cup and, holding the cup close to the skillet, slip the egg into the skillet; repeat with the remaining eggs. Reduce the heat to low; cook slowly, spooning the butter over the eggs to baste them and turning the eggs to cook on both sides, until the egg whites are completely set and the egg yolks begin to thicken but are not hard.

3. Place an egg on each plate. Spoon 2 tablespoons tomato sauce over each. Top with some sour cream, sprinkle with cilantro, and garnish with avocado slices. Serve with the remaining tomato sauce.

SERVES 4: About 310 calories, 9g protein, 13g carbohydrates, 25g fat (9g saturated), 5g fiber, 508mg sodium.

TIP

The best way to tell if an avocado is ripe is to gently squeeze the base of the fruit in the palm of your hand. It should still be firm yet yield to gentle pressure. To ripen an avocado, place it inside a brown paper bag with a couple of pieces of fruit, like a banana or apple. The fruits naturally exchange ethylene gases inside the bag, which causes them both to ripen. Once ripe, refrigerate the avocado.

Chive & Goat Cheese Frittata

Frittatas are a keto-dieter's ace in the hole: great ratios, do-ahead, delicious hot, cold, or at room temperature. And you can keep them in the fridge for a few days!

PREP: 15 MINUTES   TOTAL: 35 MINUTES

8 large eggs

⅓ cup whole milk

½ teaspoon kosher salt

⅛ teaspoon ground black pepper

1 ripe medium tomato, chopped

2 tablespoons snipped fresh chives

1 tablespoon butter or olive oil

1 package (3½ ounces) goat cheese

1. Preheat the oven to 375°F. In a medium bowl and using a wire whisk, beat the eggs, milk, salt, and pepper until well blended. Stir in the tomato and chives.

2. In a 10-inch oven-safe nonstick skillet, melt the butter over medium heat. Pour in the egg mixture. Drop tablespoons of goat cheese on top of the egg mixture and cook, without stirring, until the egg mixture begins to set around the edge, 3 to 4 minutes.

3. Place the skillet in the oven; bake until the frittata is set, 8 to 10 minutes. To serve, loosen the frittata from the skillet and slide onto a warm platter; cut into 4 wedges.

SERVES 4: About 260 calories, 18g protein, 4g carbohydrates, 19g fat (9g saturated), 0g fiber, 552mg sodium.

FUN FILLINGS

Asparagus & Romano Frittata

Prepare the egg mixture as directed, but omit the tomato, chives, and goat cheese. Trim and cut **1 pound asparagus** into 1-inch pieces. Thinly slice **4 green onions**. Melt the butter in a 10-inch nonstick skillet over medium-high heat. Stir in the asparagus; cook 4 minutes. Reduce the heat to medium; add the green onions, cook 2 minutes, stirring. Spread the vegetable mixture in the skillet. Stir **½ cup freshly grated Pecorino Romano cheese** into the eggs and pour them into the skillet. Cook as directed.

SERVES 4: About 270 calories, 21g protein, 5g carbohydrates, 18g fat (8g saturated), 2g fiber, 684mg sodium.

TIP

If your skillet is not oven-safe, wrap the handle with a double layer of foil before placing the skillet in the oven.

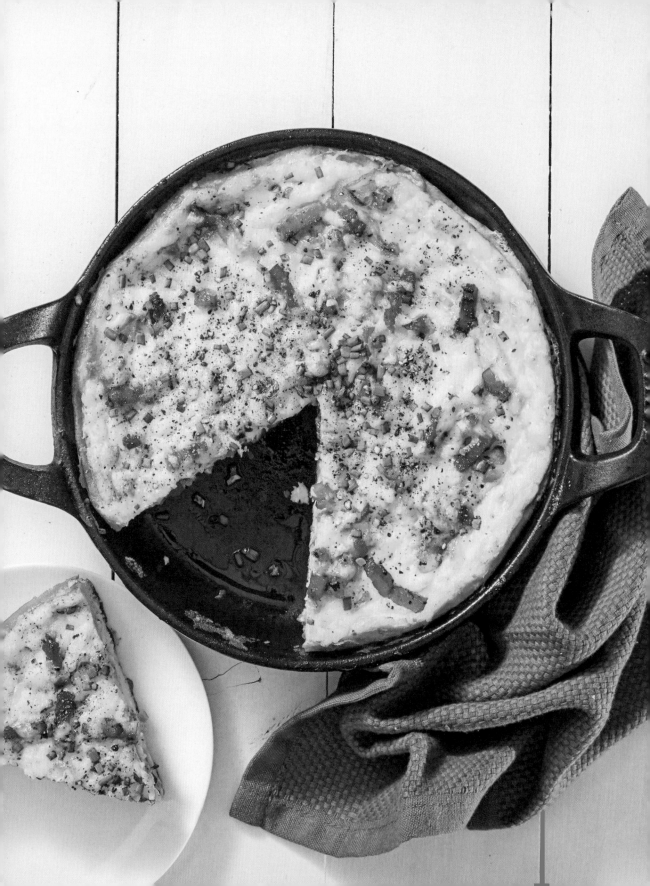

Crustless Quiche Lorraine

Bacon, shallots, and Gruyère cheese make this a craveable classic. You'll get all of the flavor without the carbs—in 20 minutes!

PREP: 12 MINUTES   TOTAL: 20 MINUTES

1 tablespoon olive oil

3 slices thick-cut bacon, chopped

1 medium shallot, thinly sliced

6 large eggs

¼ cup whole milk

⅛ teaspoon kosher salt

⅛ teaspoon ground black pepper

1 cup shredded Gruyère cheese

Chopped fresh chives, for garnish

Green salad, for serving

1. Preheat the oven to 375°F.

2. In an 8-inch oven-safe nonstick skillet, heat the oil on medium.

3. Add the bacon and shallot and cook 6 minutes, stirring occasionally.

4. In a large bowl, combine the eggs, milk, salt, and pepper and whisk until blended. Stir in the cheese.

5. Add the egg mixture to the skillet with the bacon and shallots. Cook 3 minutes, stirring occasionally to form curds and allowing the runny mixture to flow to the bottom of the pan.

6. Transfer the skillet to the oven. Bake for 8 minutes, or until the top is set.

7. Remove from the oven and garnish with chives. Serve with green salad.

SERVES 4: About 270 calories, 21g protein, 5g carbohydrates, 18g fat (8g saturated), 2g fiber, 684mg sodium.

TIP

To chop bacon easily, use kitchen shears to snip through the fatty meat.

Berry Blast Smoothie

Be sure to read the labels when buying protein powder as some have added sugars or enough carbs to send you out of ketosis.

TOTAL: 5 MINUTES

⅓ cup fresh or frozen raspberries

½ cup unsweetened canned coconut milk

1 tablespoon protein powder

1 tablespoon ground flax

8 drops stevia

½ cup ice (4 cubes)

¼ cup water

1. Put the raspberries, coconut milk, protein powder, flax, stevia, ice, and water in blender and blend until smooth.

2. Pour into a glass and serve immediately.

SERVES 1: About 335 calories, 16g protein, 11g carbohydrates, 28g fat (22g saturated), 5g fiber, 40mg sodium.

TIP

Switch up your smoothie by subbing in ⅓ cup of blueberries, blackberries, or chopped strawberries for the raspberries. Or blend a mix of your favorites together.

Lemon Cheesecake Smoothie

Yes, cheesecake for breakfast! This sweet-tart delight
spiked with ginger is an indulgent start to any day.

¾ cup unsweetened almond milk

4 tablespoons cream cheese

1 teaspoon grated lemon zest

1½ tablespoons freshly squeezed
   lemon juice

½ teaspoon grated fresh ginger

8 drops stevia

1 tablespoon protein powder

½ cup ice (4 cubes)

1. Put the almond milk, cream cheese, lemon
zest, lemon juice, ginger, stevia, protein powder,
and ice in a blender and blend until smooth.

2. Pour into a glass and serve immediately.

SERVES 1: About 295 calories, 16g protein,
8g carbohydrates, 23g fat (12g saturated),
2g fiber, 341mg sodium.

TIP

Swap in lime zest (use ½ teaspoon) and juice
if you like.

Green Light Juice

This is our kind of "juice." A savory powerhouse that blends in the solids,
so you get more fiber. Avocado adds silky texture and some healthy fat.

¾ cup unsweetened canned coconut milk

½ small (6-ounce) avocado

1 cup baby spinach

1 tablespoon fresh lime juice

1 tablespoon protein powder

¾ cup ice (6 cubes)

½ teaspoon matcha green tea powder
   (optional)

1. Put the coconut milk, avocado, spinach, lime
juice, protein powder, ice, and matcha powder
in a blender and blend until smooth.

2. Pour into a glass and serve immediately.

SERVES 1: About 505 calories, 18g protein,
14g carbohydrates, 46g fat (34g saturated),
6g fiber, 93mg sodium.

FRICO CUPS WITH GRAPE TOMATO, OLIVE & FETA SALAD (PAGES 35 & 36)

2 | Appetizers & Snacks

Snacking is the perfect way to get your ratios where you need them. Craving some crunch? Frico Cups or smaller crisps are yummy eaten alone, topped with Grape Tomato, Olive & Feta Salad or dipped in Hot 'n' Smoky Ricotta or Artichoke Dip.

Eggs are a keto mainstay and not just for breakfast. Hard cook a bunch for snacks or whip up one of our deviled favorites like Pimiento Cheese, Guacamole, or Caesar.

Fat Bombs are especially helpful in getting your ratios up. We've got your cravings covered. Smoky Manchego, Sesame Smoked Salmon, and Bacon Cheddar offer savory satisfaction. Or try the Everything Cheese Balls—no bagel needed. Sweet bombs? Yes, Chocolate Pudding, Peanut Butter, or Coconut Lime Cheesecake are your new truffles.

Tomato & Mozzarella Bites	35
Grape Tomato, Olive & Feta Salad	35
Frico Cups	36
Veggie Rolls	37
Cauliflower "Popcorn"	39
Artichoke Dip	40
Marinated Mixed Olives	40
Hot 'N' Smoky Ricotta	41
Everything Cheese Balls	43
Pimiento-Cheese Deviled Eggs	44
Sesame Smoked Salmon Bombs	46
Smoky Manchego Bombs	47
Bacon Cheddar Bombs	48
Peanut Butter Bombs	49
Chocolate Pudding Bombs	50
Coconut Lime Cheesecake Bombs	51

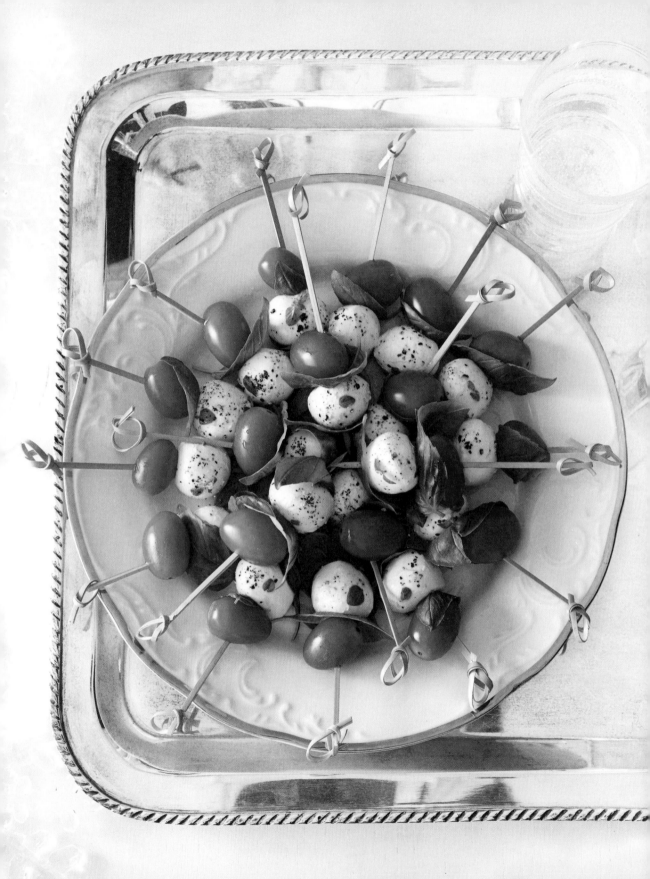

Tomato & Mozzarella Bites

Mozzarella is a perfect keto popper. Dressed with a little balsamic, tomato, and basil, it's a party!

TOTAL: 15 MINUTES

2 tablespoons olive oil

2 tablespoons white balsamic vinegar

¼ teaspoon dried oregano

¼ teaspoon kosher salt

¼ teaspoon ground black pepper

20 mini fresh mozzarella balls (ciliegini)

20 grape tomatoes

40 basil leaves

In a large bowl, whisk the oil, vinegar, oregano, salt, and pepper. Add the mozzarella balls, tossing to coat. Thread the mozzarella onto skewers, alternating with grape tomatoes and basil leaves.

SERVES 20: About 95 calories, 5g protein, 1g carbohydrates, 8g fat (4g saturated), 0g fiber, 45mg sodium.

Grape Tomato, Olive & Feta Salad

Serve in a Frico cup (page 36) or use to top grilled fish or chicken. See photo on page 32.

TOTAL: 15 MINUTES

4 cups grape tomatoes, halved

¼ cup sliced pitted green olives

⅓ cup crumbled feta cheese

1 tablespoon sherry vinegar

1 tablespoon extra-virgin olive oil

Kosher salt and ground black pepper

Fresh basil, for garnish

In a medium bowl, combine the grape tomatoes, olives, feta, sherry vinegar, and oil. Season to taste with salt and pepper. Garnish with basil. Serve in Frico Cups (page 36) or as desired.

SERVES 4: About 100 calories, 3g protein, 7g carbohydrates, 8g fat (3g saturated), 2g fiber, 240mg sodium.

Frico Cups

A yummy snack on their own or shaped into a muffin cup to fill with salad. Or make them larger and use as a wrap! See photo on page 32.

PREP: 20 MINUTES   TOTAL: 40 MINUTES

6 ounces Parmesan cheese, coarsely grated (1½ cups)

1. Preheat the oven to 375°F. Line a large baking sheet with a silicone bakeware liner. Drop 3 level tablespoons of Parmesan cheese 3 inches apart onto the baking sheet; spread it out to form rounds.

2. Bake until the edges just begin to color, 6 to 7 minutes. Use a thin metal spatula to quickly transfer each round to a muffin pan, pressing lightly in the centers. Cool before filling.

SERVES 24: About 30 calories, 3g protein, 0g carbohydrates, 2g fat (1g saturated), 0g fiber, 115mg sodium.

Parmesan Crisps

Arrange tablespoonfuls of **grated Parmesan cheese** on a silicone bakeware liner 2 inches apart. Bake 6 minutes per batch. Transfer the crisps, still on a bakeware liner, to a wire rack; cool 2 minutes. Transfer to paper towels to drain. Repeat with the remaining Parmesan.

SERVES 6: About 120 calories, 12g protein, 0g carbohydrates, 8g fat (4g saturated), 0g fiber, 460mg sodium.

Cheddar Crisps

Prepare as directed above but substitute **6 ounces sharp Cheddar cheese**, coarsely shredded (1½ cups) for the Parmesan. Bake until bubbling but not browned, 6 to 7 minutes per batch.

SERVES 6: About 120 calories, 7g protein, 0g carbohydrates, 9g fat (6g saturated), 0g fiber, 176mg sodium.

> **TIP**
>
> Frico (pronounced "FREE-koh") is what Italians call the wafer-like crisp that forms when you bake or fry shredded cheese.

Veggie Rolls

These garden-fresh snacks are a party delight—and keto-friendly, too! The rolls can stand at room temperature for up to 1 hour.

~~~~~~

TOTAL: 10 MINUTES

~~~~~~

4 zucchini or yellow squash

8 ounces cream cheese, softened

⅛ teaspoon salt

Flavorings, veggies, and/or fruits

1. With a vegetable peeler, peel the squash into wide ribbons.

2. Mix the cream cheese and salt with flavorings.

3. Cut vegetables and fruits into 2-inch-long matchsticks. Spread 1 tablespoon flavored cream cheese on one end of veggie ribbon. Add veggie/fruit sticks and roll each tightly into a bundle. Make up to 1 hour ahead; let stand at room temperature.

FUN FLAVORS

Red Pepper–Basil

Mix **½ cup roasted red peppers**, finely chopped, into the cream cheese. Serve with **basil**, **bell peppers**, and **green apples**.

SERVES 1: About 65 calories, 1g protein, 4g carbohydrates, 5g fat (3g saturated), 1g fiber, 80mg sodium.

Asian Garden

Mix **1 tablespoon soy sauce** and **2 teaspoons fresh lime juice** into the cream cheese. Roll with **radishes**, **green onions**, and **carrots**.

SERVES 1: About 55 calories, 1g protein, 3g carbohydrates, 5g fat (3g saturated), 1g fiber, 131mg sodium.

Veggie Chili

Mix **½ cup shredded Cheddar cheese** and **1 teaspoon chili powder** into the cream cheese. Roll with **cilantro**, **cucumber**, and **jicama**.

SERVES 1: About 75 calories, 2g protein, 3g carbohydrates, 6g fat (4g saturated), 1g fiber, 93mg sodium.

Zippy Pear

Mix **1 ½ tablespoons bottled horseradish** and **1 tablespoon snipped fresh chives** into the cream cheese. Roll with **parsley**, **pears**, and **celery**.

SERVES 1: About 60 calories, 1g protein, 4g carbohydrates, 5g fat (3g saturated), 1g fiber, 78mg sodium.

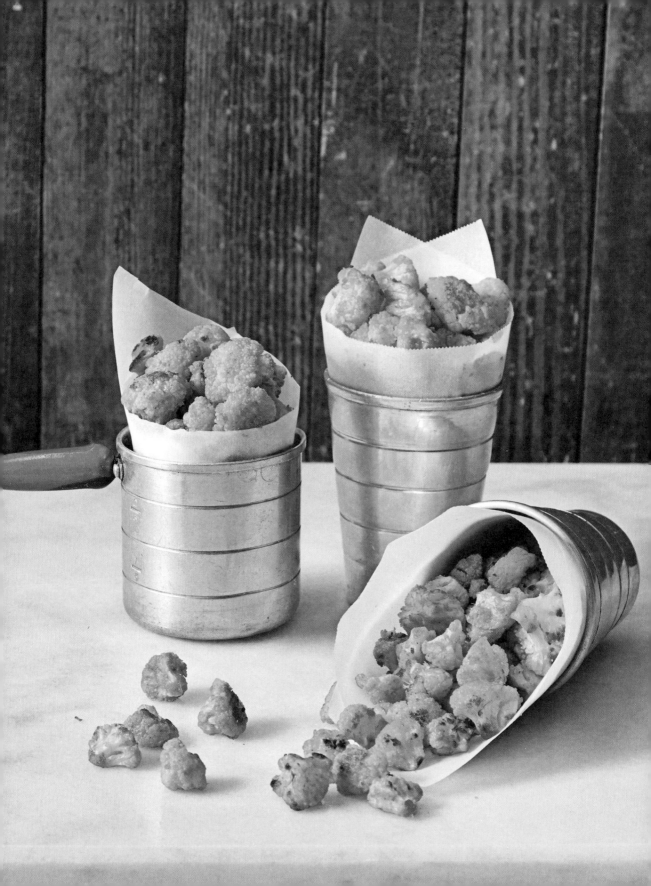

Cauliflower "Popcorn"

This satisfying take on a favorite snack is a cinch to make—and you can customize with one of our variations or your favorite spice blend.

PREP: 10 MINUTES   TOTAL: 40 MINUTES

8 cups small cauliflower florets (about 1¼ pounds), stems trimmed

3 tablespoons olive oil

¼ cup grated Parmesan cheese

1 teaspoon garlic powder

½ teaspoon ground turmeric

½ teaspoon kosher salt

1. Preheat the oven to 475°F.

2. On a large rimmed baking sheet, toss the cauliflower florets with oil, Parmesan, garlic powder, turmeric, and salt. Roast 25 to 30 minutes, or until browned and tender. Serve immediately.

SERVES 6: About 110 calories, 4g protein, 8g carbohydrates, 8g fat (2g saturated), 3g fiber, 267mg sodium.

FUN FLAVORS

Truffle

Omit the Parmesan, garlic powder, and turmeric. Toss the roasted cauliflower with **2 tablespoons truffle butter** and **½ teaspoon ground black pepper** before serving.

SERVES 6: About 120 calories, 2g protein, 5g carbohydrates, 10g fat (3g saturated), 2g fiber, 189mg sodium.

Chili Lime

Substitute **1 teaspoon chili powder** for the Parmesan and turmeric. Grate the **zest of 1 lime** over the roasted cauliflower before serving.

SERVES 6: About 90 calories, 2g protein, 5g carbohydrates, 7g fat (1g saturated), 2g fiber, 204mg sodium.

TIP

Peel and slice cauliflower stems for a crunchy snack with pesto or use them to make quick pickles.

Artichoke Dip

Lusciously creamy, try this with endive leaves or
spread it onto a piece of fish before broiling.

TOTAL: 10 MINUTES

1 lemon

1 can (13¾ ounces) artichoke hearts, drained

¼ cup mayonnaise

¼ cup freshly grated Parmesan cheese

2 tablespoons extra-virgin olive oil

1. From the lemon, grate ½ teaspoon zest
and squeeze 2 teaspoons juice.

2. In a food processor with the knife blade
attached, puree the lemon zest and juice,
artichoke hearts, mayonnaise, Parmesan, and
oil until smooth. Transfer to a serving bowl.
If you're not serving right away, cover and
refrigerate up to 3 days.

MAKES 1¼ CUPS (1 TABLESPOON SERVING): About
60 calories, 2g protein, 2g carbohydrates, 5g fat
(1g saturated), 1g fiber, 160mg sodium.

Marinated Mixed Olives

Olive oil infused with earthy notes and fresh citrus add
great flavors to these keto-friendly nibbles.

PREP: 10 MINUTES   TOTAL: 15 MINUTES, PLUS STANDING AND MARINATING

¼ cup extra-virgin olive oil

2 teaspoons fennel seeds, crushed

4 small bay leaves

2 pounds assorted Mediterranean olives,
    such as Nicoise, picholine, or Kalamata

6 strips (3 × 1 inch each) lemon peel

4 cloves garlic, crushed with the side
    of a chef's knife

1. In a 1-quart saucepan, heat the oil, fennel
seeds, and bay leaves over medium heat until
hot but not smoking. Remove the saucepan
from the heat; let stand 10 minutes.

2. In a large bowl, combine the olives, lemon
peel, garlic, and oil mixture. Cover and
refrigerate, stirring occasionally, at least 24 hours
or up to several days to blend the flavors. Store
in the refrigerator up to 1 month. Drain to serve.
(Makes about 6 cups.)

EACH ¼ CUP: About 110 calories, 1g protein,
3g carbohydrates, 10g fat (1g saturated),
1g fiber, 680mg sodium.

Hot 'N' Smoky Ricotta

Use as a dip for keto-friendly veggies—or toss with zoodles.

TOTAL: 5 MINUTES

1 cup ricotta cheese, homemade or store-bought

2 teaspoons crushed red pepper

1 teaspoon smoked paprika

Stir together the ricotta, crushed red pepper, and paprika until well blended.

EACH TABLESPOON: About 25 calories, 2g protein, 0g carbohydrates, 2g fat (1g saturated), 0g fiber, 31mg sodium.

FUN FLAVORS

Spiced Citrus

Stir together **1 cup ricotta cheese, ½ teaspoon each orange zest and ground cinnamon,** and **a few drops of stevia.**

EACH TABLESPOON: About 25 calories, 2g protein, 1g carbohydrates, 2g fat (1g saturated), 0g fiber, 13mg sodium.

Savory Herb

Stir together **1 cup ricotta cheese; 3 slices bacon,** cooked and crumbled; **1 tablespoon chopped fresh basil; 1 clove garlic,** crushed with a press; and **¼ teaspoon ground black pepper.**

EACH TABLESPOON: About 35 calories, 2g protein, 1g carbohydrates, 3g fat (1g saturated), 0g fiber, 39mg sodium.

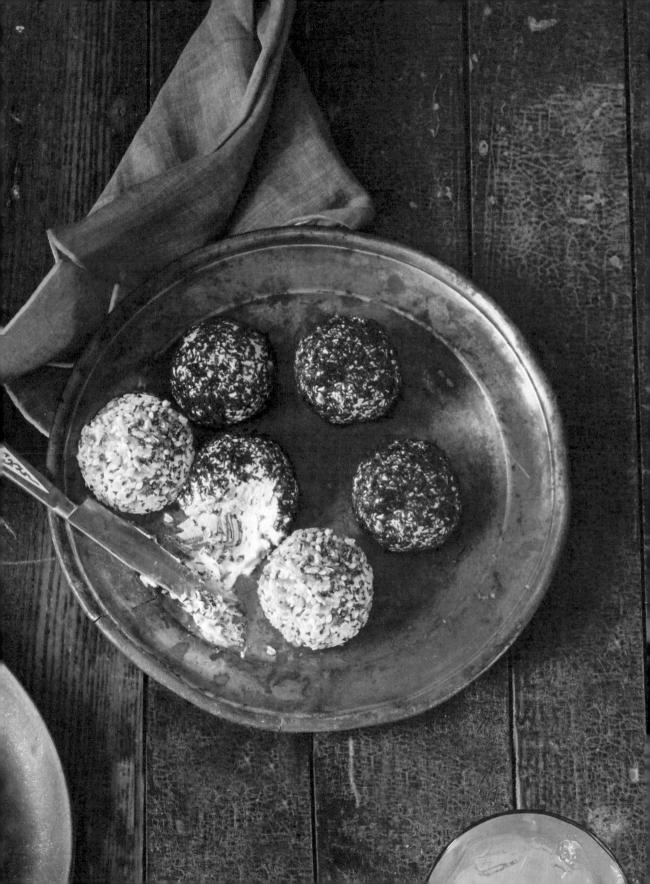

Everything Cheese Balls

These updated takes on a 50's classic get the mini treatment. Store them airtight in the fridge and they will keep for a week.

~~~~~~

TOTAL: 15 MINUTES

~~~~~~

¼ cup sesame seeds

2 tablespoons poppy seeds

2 tablespoons dried onion flakes

2 teaspoons coarsely ground black pepper

¼ teaspoon kosher salt

2 packages (8 ounces each) cream cheese, softened

In a small shallow bowl, combine the sesame seeds, poppy seeds, dried onion flakes, pepper, and salt. In a medium bowl and using a mixer, beat the cream cheese with 2 tablespoons of the seasoning mixture. Scoop and shape 2-tablespoon portions into balls. Roll them in the remaining seasoning mixture, pressing to coat.

SERVES 16: About 120 calories, 2g protein, 3g carbohydrates, 11g fat (6g saturated), 1g fiber, 120mg sodium.

FUN FLAVORS

Savory Dill

With a mixer, beat **1 package (8 ounces) cream cheese,** softened, with **1 cup crumbled feta cheese, 1 tablespoon finely chopped fresh dill,** and **2 teaspoons fresh lemon juice**. Scoop and shape 2-tablespoon portions into balls. Roll them in **3 tablespoons finely chopped fresh dill**.

SERVES 16: About 75 calories, 2g protein, 1g carbohydrates, 7g fat (4g saturated), 0g fiber, 131mg sodium.

Sweet & Spicy

With a mixer, beat **1 package (8 ounces) cream cheese** and **8 ounces softened goat cheese** until well combined. Beat in **½ teaspoon each ground cumin, ground cinnamon, ground black pepper,** and **¼ teaspoon cayenne pepper**. Scoop and shape 2-tablespoon portions into balls. Roll them in **½ cup ground pecans or walnuts**.

SERVES 16: About 105 calories, 4g protein, 1g carbohydrates, 10g fat (5g saturated), 0g fiber, 110mg sodium.

Pimiento-Cheese Deviled Eggs

We're a bit obsessed with deviled eggs. Whatever you're craving, we've got an egg for you! See photo on page 10.

See photo on page 10.

PREP: 25 MINUTES   **TOTAL: 45 MINUTES**

6 hard-cooked large eggs, peeled

3 tablespoons mayonnaise

1 teaspoon hot sauce

⅛ teaspoon kosher salt

¼ cup shredded extra-sharp
   Cheddar cheese

½ (2-ounce) jar pimientos,
   well drained and finely chopped

½ green onion, finely chopped

Paprika, for garnish

Cut the eggs in half lengthwise. Transfer the yolks to a medium bowl and mash with mayonnaise, hot sauce, and salt until almost smooth. Fold in the Cheddar, pimientos, and green onion. Spoon into the egg whites. Garnish with paprika. Serve immediately or refrigerate, covered with plastic, up to 1 day.

SERVES 6: About 140 calories, 8g protein, 1g carbohydrates, 11g fat (3g saturated), 195mg sodium.

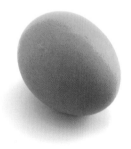

FUN FLAVORS

Ham & Cheese

Mash **6 hard-cooked yolks** with ¼ cup **mayonnaise**; ¼ cup finely grated sharp Cheddar **cheese**; 1 tablespoon sweet relish, drained; **1 slice deli ham**, finely chopped; ½ **tablespoon spicy brown mustard**; and ⅛ teaspoon kosher salt.

SERVES 6: About 165 calories, 8g protein, 2g carbohydrates, 14g fat (4g saturated), 0g fiber, 283mg sodium.

Guacamole

Mash **6 hard-cooked yolks** with ½ small **ripe avocado**; 2 tablespoons mayonnaise; **2 tablespoons fresh cilantro**, finely chopped; ½ **very small shallot**, finely chopped; 1 tablespoon **fresh lime juice**; and ¼ teaspoon kosher salt. Garnish the filled eggs with **thinly sliced serrano chilies**.

SERVES 6: About 130 calories, 7g protein, 2g carbohydrates, 11g fat (2g saturated), 1g fiber, 173mg sodium.

Pesto-Bacon

Mash **6 hard-cooked yolks** with ¼ cup mayonnaise, **2 tablespoons pesto**, and **1 tablespoon fresh lemon juice**. Spoon into the whites; garnish with **crumbled cooked bacon**.

SERVES 6: About 170 calories, 8g protein, 1g carbohydrates, 15g fat (3g saturated), 0g fiber, 197mg sodium.

Caesar

Mash **6 hard-cooked yolks** with **¼ cup mayonnaise, 2 tablespoons grated Parmesan cheese, 1 tablespoon fresh lemon juice, 1 teaspoon Dijon mustard**, and **½ small clove garlic**, crushed with a press. Garnish the filled eggs with **ground black pepper** and **chopped fresh basil**.

SERVES 6: About 145 calories, 7g protein, 1g carbohydrates, 13g fat (3g saturated), 0g fiber, 172mg sodium.

Miso-Ginger

Mash **6 hard-cooked yolks** with **¼ cup mayonnaise, 1 tablespoon white or yellow miso, ½ teaspoon grated peeled fresh ginger**, and **¼ teaspoon ground black pepper**. Garnish the filled eggs with **snipped fresh chives** and **finely julienned peeled fresh ginger**.

SERVES 6: About 145 calories, 7g protein, 2g carbohydrates, 12g fat (3g saturated), 0g fiber, 200mg sodium.

Crunchy Curry

Mash **6 hard-cooked yolks** with **¼ cup mayonnaise, 1 teaspoon curry powder, 1 teaspoon fresh lemon juice**, and **⅛ teaspoon kosher salt**. Spoon into the whites; garnish with **sliced almonds** and **snipped fresh chives**.

SERVES 6: About 150 calories, 7g protein, 1g carbohydrates, 13g fat (3g saturated), 0g fiber, 162mg sodium.

Classic

Mash **6 hard-cooked yolks** with **¼ cup mayonnaise, ½ tablespoon Dijon or spicy brown mustard**, and **¼ tablespoon hot sauce**. Garnish the filled eggs with **paprika**.

SERVES 6: About 140 calories, 6g protein, 1g carbohydrates, 12g fat (3g saturated), 0g fiber, 157mg sodium.

Smoky Chipotle

Mash **6 hard-cooked yolks** with **¼ cup mayonnaise, 1 tablespoon chopped chipotles in adobo, ½ teaspoon distilled white vinegar**, and **⅛ teaspoon kosher salt**. Spoon into the whites; garnish with **chili powder** and **chopped fresh cilantro**.

SERVES 6: About 140 calories, 6g protein, 1g carbohydrates, 12g fat (3g saturated), 0g fiber, 184mg sodium.

TIP

The trick to preventing that green tinge around the yolk when hard-boiling eggs? Barely boil them! Cooking eggs over too high a heat or for too long causes the yolks to produce ferrous sulfide, which leaves that telltale (though harmless) green ring. For golden yolks, place eggs in a saucepan that's large enough to fit them in a single layer; add enough cold water to cover by about an inch. Heat just to boiling; then cover the pot, remove from heat, and let it stand 14 minutes. Drain and then run cold water over the eggs in the pot until they're cool to the touch. They'll be perfect!

Sesame Smoked Salmon Bombs

Pistachios add crunch to these savory nuggets.
Swap in roasted almonds if you prefer.

~~~~~~
TOTAL: 10 MINUTES, PLUS CHILLING
~~~~~~

4 ounces cream cheese, at room temperature

¼ cup butter, at room temperature

½ teaspoon grated lemon zest

2 teaspoons fresh lemon juice

1 teaspoon toasted sesame oil

½ teaspoon ground ginger

2 ounces smoked salmon, chopped

**3 tablespoons sesame seeds or
chopped pistachios**

1. Line a baking sheet with parchment paper and set aside.

2. In a medium bowl, stir together the cream cheese, butter, lemon zest, lemon juice, sesame oil, and ginger until very well blended. Stir in the smoked salmon until combined.

3. Drop a tablespoon of the mixture on the prepared baking sheet and repeat until you have 12 equal-size mounds.

4. Place the baking sheet in the refrigerator until the bombs are firm, 1½ to 2 hours.

5. Place the sesame seeds or nuts in small, shallow dish. Using your hands, quickly shape the bombs into balls and toss them in sesame seeds to coat. Store in a sealed container in the refrigerator for up to 1 week.

SERVES 12: About 85 calories, 2g protein,
1g carbohydrates, 9g fat (5g saturated),
0g fiber, 93mg sodium.

Smoky Manchego Bombs

Spanish-style cured chorizo has a smoky flavor and is similar to pepperoni in texture. If you don't find chorizo, you could substitute with pepperoni.

TOTAL: 10 MINUTES, PLUS CHILLING

2 dried chorizo sausages, casings removed

4 ounces cubed Manchego cheese,
   at room temperature

4 ounces butter, at room temperature

2 ounces cream cheese, at room temperature

1½ teaspoons smoked paprika

½ teaspoon onion powder

1. Line a baking sheet with parchment paper and set aside.

2. In a mini food processor, finely chop the chorizo. Place it in a small, shallow dish and set aside.

3. Add the Manchego to the mini food processor and process until finely chopped. Add the butter, cream cheese, paprika, and onion powder. Process until well blended.

4. Drop a tablespoon of the mixture on the prepared baking sheet and repeat until you have 12 even mounds.

5. Place the baking sheet in the refrigerator until the bombs are firm, about 1½ hours.

6. Using your hands, quickly shape the bombs into balls and toss them in the chopped chorizo to coat. Store in a sealed container in the refrigerator for up to 1 week.

SERVES 12: About 170 calories, 5g protein, 1g carbohydrates, 16g fat (9g saturated), 0g fiber, 253mg sodium.

Bacon Cheddar Bombs

Here's proof bacon and cheddar are a winning combo. This comfort bomb gets a kick from jalapeño, which you can omit if you like.

TOTAL: 10 MINUTES, PLUS CHILLING

8 slices bacon, cooked, drained, and chopped

4 ounces cream cheese, at room temperature

½ cup shredded sharp Cheddar cheese

½ jalapeño chili, seeded and finely chopped

1. Line a baking sheet with parchment paper and set aside.

2. In a medium bowl, stir together ¼ cup of the chopped bacon, cream cheese, Cheddar, and jalapeño until well blended.

3. Drop a tablespoon of the mixture on the prepared baking sheet and repeat until you have 12 even mounds.

4. Place the baking sheet in the refrigerator until the bombs are firm, about 30 minutes.

5. Place the remaining bacon in a small, shallow dish. Using your hands, quickly shape the bombs into balls and toss them in the bacon to coat. Store in sealed container in the refrigerator up to 1 week.

SERVES 12: About 80 calories, 4g protein, 1g carbohydrates, 7g fat (3g saturated), 0g fiber, 150mg sodium.

Peanut Butter Bombs

Move over peanut butter cups! This sweet bite hits all the notes without the sugar. Be sure to use only natural unsweetened peanut butter.

TOTAL: 15 MINUTES, PLUS CHILLING

4 ounces cream cheese, at room temperature

½ cup natural peanut butter

2 tablespoons softened coconut oil

12 drops liquid stevia

⅛ teaspoon ground cinnamon

⅓ cup sugar-free dark chocolate chips

½ cup unsalted peanuts, chopped

1. Line a baking sheet with parchment paper and set aside.

2. In a medium bowl, stir together the cream cheese, peanut butter, coconut oil, stevia, and cinnamon until well blended. Stir in the chocolate chips.

3. Drop a tablespoon of the mixture on the prepared baking sheet and repeat until you have 12 even mounds.

4. Place the baking sheet in the refrigerator until the bombs are firm, about 1½ hours.

5. Place the chopped peanuts in a small, shallow dish. Using your hands, shape the bombs into balls. Roll them in chopped peanuts to coat. Store in a sealed container in the refrigerator up to 1 week.

SERVES 12: About 180 calories, 5g protein, 7g carbohydrates, 15g fat (6g saturated), 2g fiber, 66mg sodium.

Chocolate Pudding Bombs

Craving chocolate? Part truffle, part pudding, this truffle will satisfy!
You can use almond butter instead of cashew, if you like.

TOTAL: 10 MINUTES, PLUS CHILLING

¼ **cup coconut oil**

¼ **cup unsweetened cocoa**

1 **teaspoon instant espresso-coffee powder**

½ **cup cashew butter**

2 **ounces cream cheese, at room temperature**

12 **drops liquid stevia**

1. Line a baking sheet with parchment paper and set aside.

2. In a medium microwave-safe bowl, microwave the coconut oil on High 30 seconds, or until melted. Whisk in the cocoa and espresso powder until smooth. Whisk in the cashew butter, cream cheese, and stevia until smooth and well blended.

3. Drop a tablespoon of the mixture on the prepared baking sheet and repeat until you have 12 even mounds.

4. Place the baking sheet in the refrigerator until the bombs are firm, about 30 minutes.

5. Store in a sealed container in the refrigerator for up to 1 week.

SERVES 12: About 125 calories, 3g protein, 4g carbohydrates, 12g fat (6g saturated), 1g fiber, 17mg sodium.

Coconut Lime Cheesecake Bombs

Who says there is no dessert on the keto plan? Lime
and coconut make this an irresistible popper.

TOTAL: 10 MINUTES, PLUS CHILLING

⅔ cup softened coconut oil

6 tablespoons cream cheese, at room
   temperature

2 teaspoons grated lime zest

2 teaspoons fresh lime juice

8 drops liquid stevia

1 drop coconut extract or almond
   extract

7 tablespoons finely grated
   unsweetened coconut

1. Line a baking sheet with parchment paper
and set aside.

2. In a medium bowl, stir together the
coconut oil, cream cheese, lime zest, lime
juice, and stevia until very well blended. Stir
in 4 tablespoons of the grated coconut until
combined.

3. Drop a tablespoon of the mixture on the
prepared baking sheet and repeat until you
have 12 even mounds.

4. Place the baking sheet in the refrigerator
until the bombs are firm, 1 to 2 hours.

5. Place the remaining 3 tablespoons grated
coconut in a small, shallow dish. Using your
hands, quickly shape the bombs into balls and
toss them in coconut to coat. Store in a sealed
container in the refrigerator for up to 1 week.

SERVES 12: About 155 calories, 1g protein,
1g carbohydrates, 16g fat (13g saturated),
1g fiber, 24mg sodium.

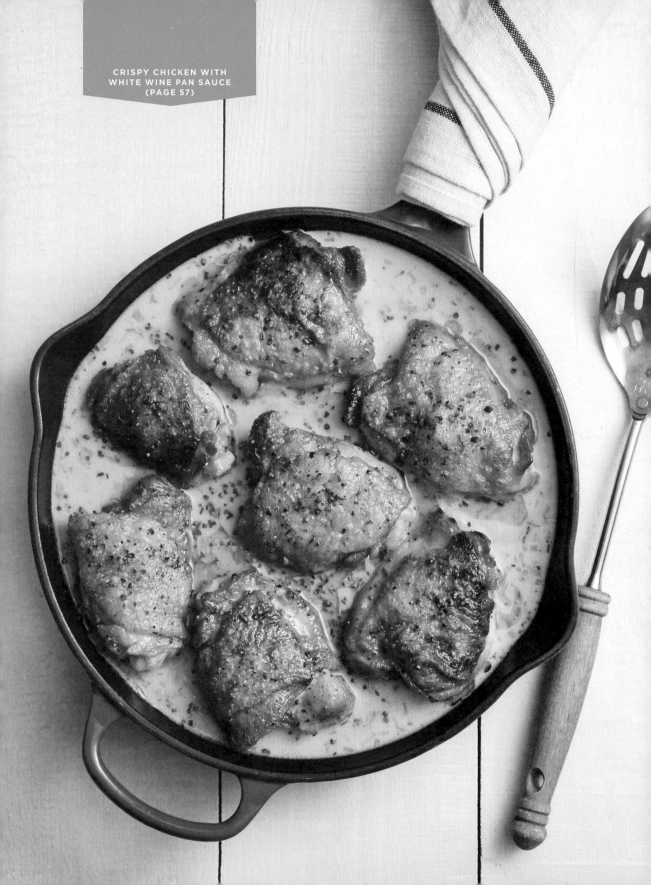

CRISPY CHICKEN WITH
WHITE WINE PAN SAUCE
(PAGE 57)

3 | Poultry

Forget boring diet chicken. This is not where we're going. What you already know is that chicken is a perfect canvas for about any main dish you want. *Good Housekeeping* has thousands of recipes to prove it. Here, we've chosen options to get you jazzed about eating chicken—and achieving your keto goals. How about draping it with pancetta and simply roasting it with green beans? Spanish Chicken & Peppers is another reason to love the simplicity of sheet pan roasting. Chicken Caprese is a quick skillet riff on the summery caprese salad of tomatoes and mozzarella.

Want a little spice? Fiery Kung Pao Chicken stirfry, Chipotle Orange Chicken, or Spicy Jerk Drumsticks deliver.

Roasted Baby Vine Tomato Grilled Chicken.................55

Nigerian Peanutty Suya Skewers.......56

Crispy Chicken with White Wine Pan Sauce.................57

Mushroom Chicken Skillet with Herbed Cream Sauce.................59

Lighter Chicken Cacciatore.................61

Chicken with Creamy Spinach & Artichokes.................62

Chicken Souvlaki Skewers.................63

Lemony Herb Roast Chicken.................65

Pancetta Chicken.................66

Spicy Jerk Drumsticks.................67

Fiery Kung Pao Chicken.................69

Glazed Bacon-Wrapped Turkey Breast.................71

Chipotle Orange Chicken.................73

Cilantro-Lime Chicken.................74

Chicken Caprese.................75

Spanish Chicken & Peppers.................77

Moroccan Chicken with Preserved Lemons & Olives.................79

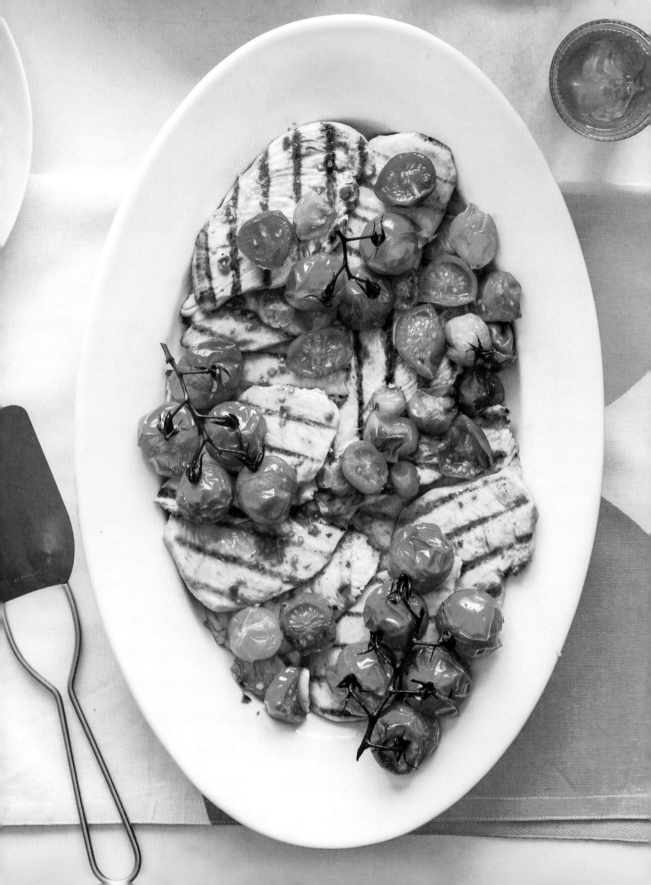

Roasted Baby Vine Tomato Grilled Chicken

Roasting the tomatoes concentrates their flavor and sweetness.
No tarragon? Mint, basil, or cilantro are delicious alternatives.

PREP: 20 MINUTES   TOTAL: 45 MINUTES

**2 pounds mixed-size cherry tomatoes,
on the vine if desired (about 4 pints)**

4 large garlic cloves, crushed

¼ cup plus 1 tablespoon extra-virgin olive oil

¼ teaspoon crushed red pepper

Kosher salt

**1½ pounds chicken breast cutlets
(about ⅓ inch thick)**

¼ teaspoon ground black pepper

1½ tablespoons chopped fresh tarragon

1. Preheat the oven to 500°F. Preheat a grill on medium-high. Cut about 1 cup of the largest tomatoes in half. On a rimmed baking sheet, toss all the tomatoes with the garlic, ¼ cup of the olive oil, crushed red pepper, and ¾ teaspoon salt.

2. Roast the tomatoes on an upper oven rack, stirring halfway through, until the tomatoes burst and soften and some are beginning to char, about 20 minutes. (If most juices have evaporated, stir in 1 to 2 tablespoons water to create more sauce.)

3. Meanwhile, coat the chicken cutlets with the remaining 1 tablespoon olive oil and season with ¼ teaspoon salt and the pepper. Grill until lightly charred and just cooked through, 2 to 3 minutes per side.

4. Gently toss the tomatoes with the chopped tarragon. Spoon the tomatoes and juices on top of chicken and serve.

SERVES 4: About 390 calories, 37g protein, 10g carbohydrates, 22g fat (4g saturated), 2g fiber, 595mg sodium.

Nigerian Peanutty Suya Skewers

Warm spices meet crunchy nuts in this yummy kebab. Serve it with a salad or Sautéed Spinach with Garlic (page 129).

~~~~~~

TOTAL: 30 MINUTES, PLUS MARINATING

~~~~~~

½ cup roasted unsalted peanuts

1 teaspoon ground ginger

1 teaspoon garlic powder

1 teaspoon onion powder

½ teaspoon ground cinnamon

½ teaspoon cayenne pepper

½ teaspoon kosher salt

½ teaspoon ground black pepper

1 tablespoon canola oil

1 pound beef sirloin, thinly sliced

2 limes, halved

1. In a food processor, pulse the peanuts with the spices, salt, and black pepper until finely chopped (do not let it become a paste). Add the oil and pulse to combine.

2. In a bowl, toss the beef in the peanut mixture making sure to coat the meat evenly. Cover; refrigerate at least 1 hour or up to overnight.

3. Preheat the grill on medium-high. Thread the beef onto skewers and grill until charred, 2 to 3 minutes per side. Squeeze lime halves over the top, then transfer to a platter and serve.

SERVES 4: About 330 calories, 29g protein, 8g carbohydrates, 21g fat (5g saturated), 2g fiber, 295mg sodium.

Crispy Chicken with White Wine Pan Sauce

Skillet and sheet pan get this dinner on the table fast. For an easy side, toss a pound of trimmed asparagus with a tablespoon of oil and roast along with the chicken for 10 minutes. See photo on page 52.

PREP: 15 MINUTES   TOTAL: 30 MINUTES

2 teaspoons olive oil

2½ pounds chicken thighs

Kosher salt

2 medium shallots, chopped

⅔ cup white wine

¼ teaspoon dried rosemary

3 tablespoons sour cream

½ cup chicken broth

Snipped fresh chives, for garnish

1. Preheat the oven to 450°F. Line a rimmed baking sheet with aluminum foil.

2. In a 12-inch skillet, heat the oil on medium-high. Season the chicken thighs with ½ teaspoon salt and place in the skillet, skin sides down. Cook 6 to 8 minutes, or until browned. Transfer the chicken to the prepared baking sheet, skin sides up. Roast 15 minutes, or until cooked through (165°F).

3. Meanwhile, to the same skillet on medium, add the shallots. Cook 2 minutes. Add the white wine, rosemary, and ¼ teaspoon salt. Simmer 2 minutes, scraping up the browned bits. Whisk in the sour cream and broth.

4. Serve the chicken with the sauce, garnished with snipped chives.

SERVES 4: About 465 calories, 40g protein, 4g carbohydrates, 31g fat (9g saturated), 1g fiber, 615mg sodium.

SEAR & DEGLAZE

- Use a 12-inch skillet so the food will have plenty of room to brown, not steam.

- Pat your protein dry with a paper towel. Liquid interferes with searing.

- Season it right. Sprinkle your meat on both sides with 1/4 teaspoon each kosher salt and ground black pepper (for 4 servings).

- Get your oil nice and hot on medium-high heat. It should ripple slightly before you add the meat. Once meat is in the pan, don't move it until it releases easily.

- Choose the right tool. After adding liquid to the pan to deglaze, use a wooden spoon to scrape up all the tasty browned bits.

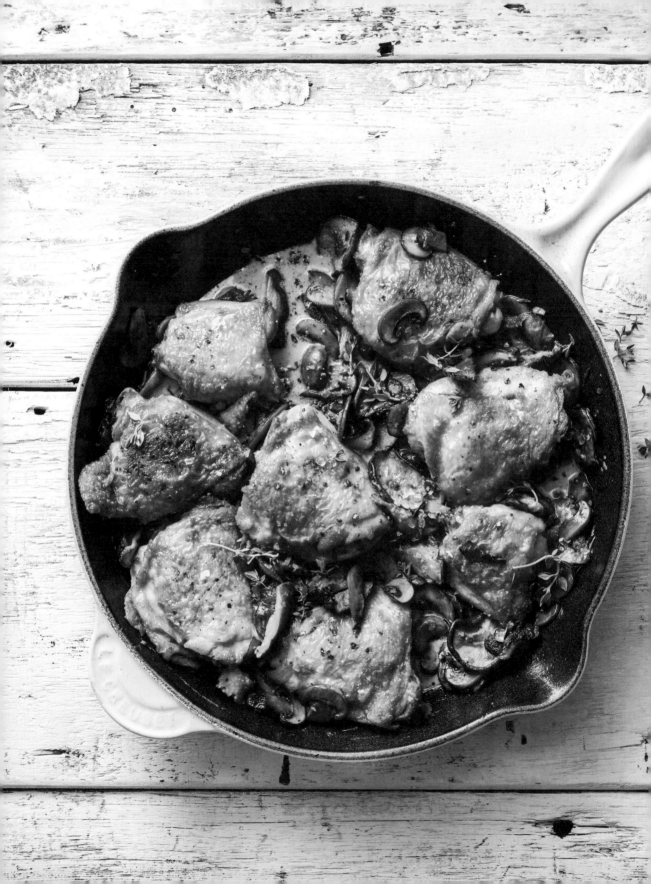

Mushroom Chicken Skillet with Herbed Cream Sauce

This classic French dish gets a twist with the addition of shitake mushrooms. If they're not in your market you can use all creminis.

PREP: 20 MINUTES   **TOTAL: 45 MINUTES**

1 tablespoon butter

3 tablespoons olive oil, divided

10 ounces cremini mushrooms, sliced

8 ounces shiitake mushrooms, stems removed and discarded and caps sliced

Kosher salt

1 large shallot, finely chopped

8 small chicken thighs (about 2 pounds)

¼ teaspoon ground black pepper

⅓ cup dry white wine

½ cup low-sodium chicken broth

3 sprigs thyme, plus more (optional) for garnish

¼ cup heavy cream

1. Preheat the oven to 375°F. In a large oven-safe skillet, heat butter and 2 tablespoons of the oil on medium-high. Once the butter foams, add the mushrooms and a pinch of salt and cook, tossing occasionally, for 5 minutes. Add the shallot and cook, tossing occasionally, until the mushrooms are golden brown, 2 to 3 minutes; transfer to plate and wipe the skillet clean.

2. Return the skillet to medium heat. Rub the chicken with the remaining 1 tablespoon oil and season with ¼ teaspoon salt and the pepper. Add chicken to skillet, skin side down, and cook until browned, 10 to 12 minutes; drain any excess fat. Turn the chicken over; add the wine, broth, and thyme sprigs. Transfer the skillet to the oven until the chicken is cooked through (165°F), 5 to 6 minutes.

3. Transfer the chicken to a plate, discard the thyme, and return the skillet to medium heat. Stir in the cream and mushroom mixture and cook until heated through, about 2 minutes. Serve with chicken. Garnish with thyme, if desired.

SERVES 4: About 605 calories, 46g protein, 9g carbohydrates, 44g fat (14g saturated), 2g fiber, 370mg sodium.

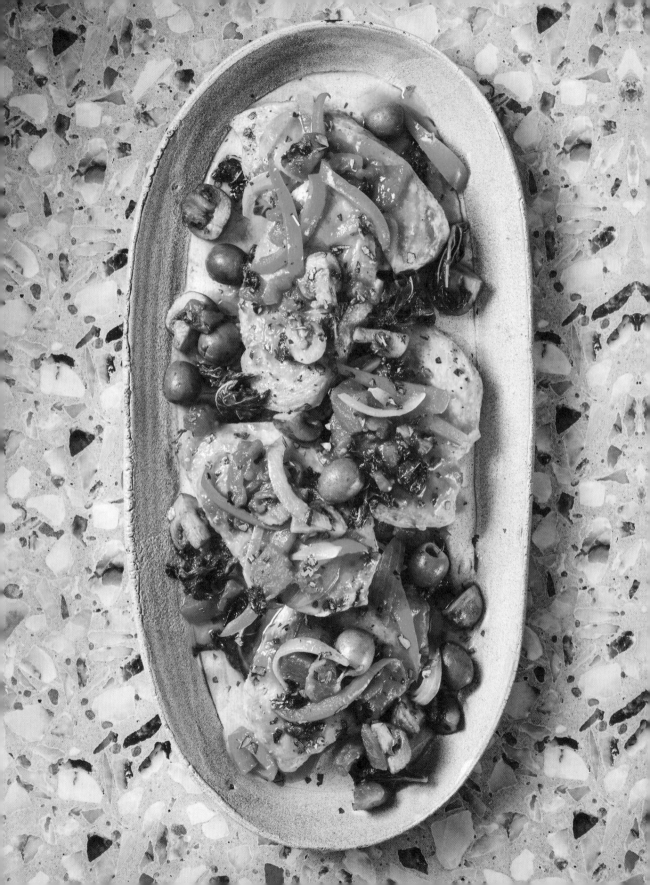

Lighter Chicken Cacciatore

Mushrooms add satisfying umami to dishes and are excellent sources of potassium and selenium as well as a plant-based source of Vitamin D.

PREP: 30 MINUTES   TOTAL: 50 MINUTES

2 tablespoons olive oil

6 small boneless, skinless chicken breasts (5 ounces each)

½ teaspoon kosher salt

½ teaspoon ground black pepper

10 ounces cremini mushrooms, quartered

1 small onion, thinly sliced

1 red bell pepper, thinly sliced

2 cloves garlic, finely chopped

2 teaspoons fresh rosemary, finely chopped

1 bay leaf

¾ cup dry white wine

1 can (28 ounces) diced tomatoes

8 ounces kale, stems discarded and leaves chopped

½ cup pitted green olives

¼ cup flat-leaf parsley, chopped

1. In a large deep skillet, heat the oil on medium-high. Season the chicken with the salt and pepper and cook until golden brown, 3 to 4 minutes per side; transfer to a plate and cover to keep warm.

2. Add the mushrooms to the skillet and cook, tossing occasionally, until golden brown and tender, about 4 minutes. Transfer to the plate with the chicken.

3. Lower the heat to medium. Add the onion, bell pepper, garlic, rosemary, and bay leaf and cook, stirring occasionally, until tender, 8 to 10 minutes. Add the wine and cook, stirring and scraping up browned bits, until reduced by half, about 3 minutes. Stir in the tomatoes (and their juices).

4. Return the chicken and mushrooms to the skillet, nestling the chicken in the tomatoes, cover, and simmer for 15 minutes. Fold in the kale, cover, and cook 10 to 12 minutes more. Uncover, discard the bay leaf, stir in the olives and parsley, and serve.

SERVES 6: About 300 calories, 36g protein, 15g carbohydrates, 10g fat (1.5g saturated), 3g fiber, 690mg sodium.

Chicken with Creamy Spinach & Artichokes

You'll love this sophisticated take on spinach and artichoke dip. If you want to use frozen artichokes, thaw them and cook for a minute or 2 longer.

PREP: 10 MINUTES   TOTAL: 30 MINUTES

4 boneless, skinless chicken breasts (6 ounces each)

Kosher salt and ground black pepper

Olive oil

Juice of 1 lemon

1 can (14 ounces) artichoke hearts, drained and halved lengthwise

2 cloves garlic, thinly sliced

½ cup dry white wine

¼ cup sour cream

1 bunch spinach leaves, stems removed and discarded

1. Season the chicken breasts with ½ teaspoon each salt and pepper. In a skillet on medium, heat 1 tablespoon oil and cook the chicken 6 to 8 minutes per side. Remove from heat and drizzle the lemon juice on top.

2. In the same skillet, heat 1 tablespoon oil on medium-high and brown the artichoke hearts, cut sides down, about 3 minutes.

3. Lower the heat to medium; add the garlic to the artichoke hearts and toss. Stir in the white wine; cook 2 minutes. Stir in the sour cream and spinach leaves; season with salt and pepper and cook until just wilted.

SERVES 4: About 305 calories, 38g protein, 10g carbohydrates, 11.5g fat (3g saturated), 2g fiber, 675mg sodium.

Chicken Souvlaki Skewers

Bold Mediterranean flavors star in this easy chicken dish. You can use a grill pan or your broiler for the chicken if it's not grilling weather.

PREP: 15 MINUTES   TOTAL: 25 MINUTES

1 pound boneless, skinless chicken breasts, cut into 1-inch chunks

3 tablespoons olive oil, divided

½ teaspoon ground coriander

½ teaspoon dried oregano

Kosher salt and ground black pepper

1 pint grape tomatoes

2 cloves garlic, chopped

3 tablespoons fresh lemon juice, divided, plus lemon wedges for serving

½ head romaine lettuce, shredded

4 green onions, thinly sliced

½ cup dill, chopped

1. Preheat the grill on medium-high. Toss the chicken with 1 tablespoon of the oil, then add the coriander, oregano, and ¼ teaspoon each salt and pepper and toss. Thread the chicken onto skewers.

2. Place the tomatoes and garlic on a large piece of heavy-duty foil. Sprinkle with 1 tablespoon of the oil and ¼ teaspoon each salt and pepper. Fold and crimp the foil to form a pouch.

3. Place the pouch and skewers on the grill. Cook, shaking the pouch and turning the skewers occasionally, until the chicken is cooked through, 8 to 10 minutes. Just before removing it from the grill, brush the chicken with 1 tablespoon of the lemon juice.

4. Meanwhile, in a bowl, toss the lettuce, onions, and dill with the remaining 2 tablespoons lemon juice, 1 tablespoon oil, and ¼ teaspoon each salt and pepper.

5. Serve the chicken, tomatoes, and salad with lemon wedges.

SERVES 4: About 245 calories, 25g protein, 8g carbohydrates, 13g fat (2g saturated), 3g fiber, 426mg sodium.

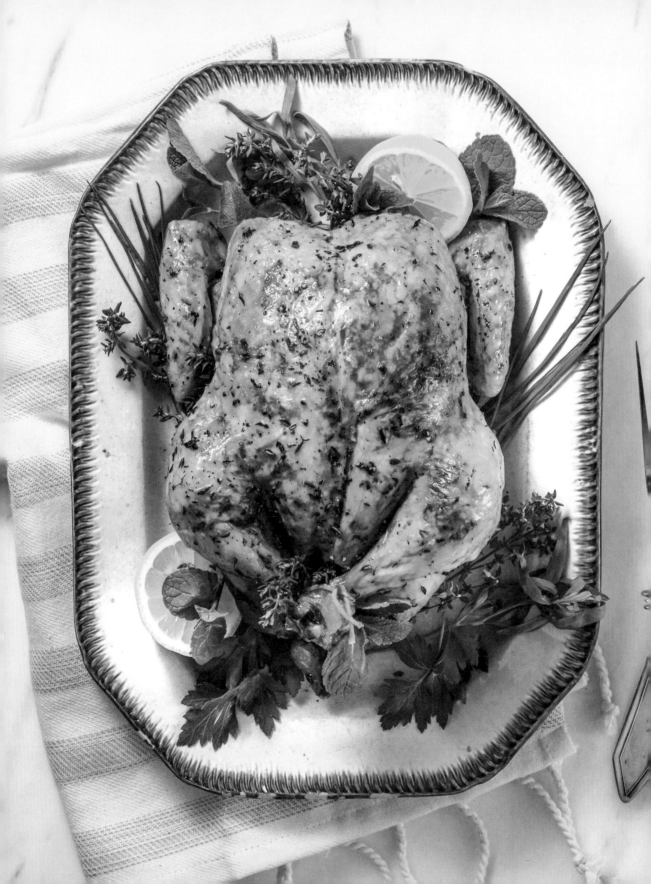

Lemony Herb Roast Chicken

Better than rotisserie and almost as easy. The sweet roasted radishes are perfect with the lemony meat. Use any leftover chicken for the Buffalo Chicken Cobb (page 136).

PREP: 15 MINUTES   TOTAL: 1 HOUR 20 MINUTES

2 teaspoons finely grated lemon zest

2 cloves garlic, crushed with a press

1 teaspoon fresh thyme, chopped

4 tablespoons butter, divided, softened

Kosher salt and ground black pepper

1 whole chicken (4 to 5 pounds), patted dry

1 medium onion, thinly sliced

1 bunch radishes, trimmed and quartered

¼ cup water

1. Preheat the oven to 350°F.

2. In a bowl, mash together the lemon zest, garlic, thyme, 2 tablespoons of the butter, and ½ teaspoon each salt and pepper until combined. With your fingers, gently separate the skin from the breast and thighs of the chicken. Spread the butter mixture evenly under the skin. Tie the drumsticks together and tuck the wings behind breast.

3. Place the chicken on rack fitted into medium roasting pan. Arrange the onion and radishes around the chicken. Melt the remaining 2 tablespoons butter; brush it all over chicken, then sprinkle with ½ teaspoon each salt and pepper. Pour the water into bottom of the roasting pan.

4. Roast the chicken 50 minutes. Raise the oven temperature to 425°F and roast, checking to make sure the water has not completely evaporated (add another ¼ cup, if necessary), for 15 to 20 minutes, or until a thermometer inserted into thickest part of thigh registers 165°F.

5. Let the chicken rest at least 15 minutes before carving and serving.

SERVES 6: 415 calories 40g protein, 1g carbohydrates, 27g fat (10g saturated), 0g fiber, 345mg sodium.

Pancetta Chicken

Sheet pans are a boon to any weeknight cook, and are especially keto-friendly. You can cook your protein and a veggie side at the same time with about 10 minutes of prep.

PREP: 10 MINUTES   TOTAL: 40 MINUTES

4 small skinless, boneless chicken breast halves (about 1½ pounds)

Kosher salt and ground black pepper

4 slices pancetta

1 pound green beans

2 teaspoons olive oil

Lemon wedges, for serving

1. Preheat the oven to 450°F. Line a rimmed baking sheet with foil.

2. Sprinkle the chicken breast halves with ½ teaspoon salt; drape pancetta over each piece, tucking the ends under. Sprinkle lightly with pepper. Place on the prepared baking sheet.

3. On another baking sheet, toss the green beans with the oil; season with salt and pepper.

4. Roast the chicken and green beans 30 minutes, or until the chicken is cooked through (165°F). Serve the chicken and green beans together with lemon wedges.

SERVES 4: About 265 calories, 38g protein, 10g carbohydrates, 8g fat (2g saturated), 4g fiber, 520mg sodium

Spicy Jerk Drumsticks

Serve these spicy legs with a side of cauliflower rice.
If you're spice shy, reduce jalapenos to one.

PREP: 15 MINUTES   TOTAL: 55 MINUTES, PLUS MARINATING

¼ **cup olive oil**

¼ **cup soy sauce**

3 **tablespoons fresh lime juice**

5 **thin slices peeled fresh ginger**

3 **green onions, sliced**

2 **cloves garlic**

3 **jalapeño chilies, or 1 habanero chili**

5 **sprigs fresh thyme**

¼ **teaspoon ground allspice**

¾ **teaspoon salt**

12 **chicken drumsticks**

**Sliced jalapeño chilies and lime wedges,
  for garnish (optional)**

1. In a blender, puree the oil, soy sauce, lime juice, ginger, green onions, garlic, chilies, thyme, allspice, and salt until smooth; transfer to gallon-size resealable bag along with the chicken. Seal the bag, removing excess air. Toss well to coat the chicken; place the bag on a large plate. Refrigerate at least 4 hours or up to overnight.

2. Preheat the oven to 425°F. Line a large rimmed baking sheet with foil; fit a wire rack in the baking sheet. Remove the drumsticks from the marinade (discard marinade) and gently pat them dry with paper towels; arrange them on the rack, spaced 1 inch apart. Roast 35 to 40 minutes, or until cooked through (160°F). Garnish with jalapeños and lime wedges, if desired.

SERVES 6: About 195 calories, 21g protein, 2g carbohydrates, 11g fat (3g saturated), 0g fiber, 300mg sodium.

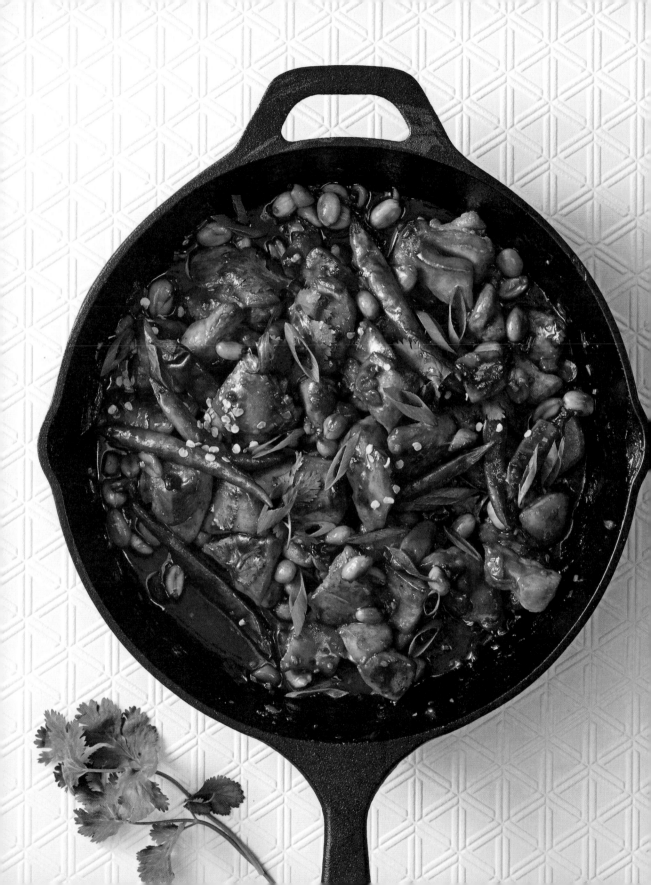

Fiery Kung Pao Chicken

The dried chiles de árbol pack a punch. If you can't find them
in your market, use ½ teaspoon ground cayenne.

PREP: 15 MINUTES   TOTAL: 30 MINUTES, PLUS MARINATING

¼ cup unsweetened rice wine

¼ cup soy sauce

1 tablespoon cornstarch

1½ pounds skinless, boneless chicken thighs,
   trimmed and cut into scant 1-inch chunks

1 tablespoon vegetable oil

1 bunch green onions, thinly sliced

3 cloves garlic, chopped

2 tablespoons finely chopped peeled fresh
   ginger

½ cup roasted unsalted peanuts

3 tablespoons balsamic vinegar

8 whole dried chilies de árbol

Chopped fresh cilantro, for garnish

1. In a medium bowl, whisk together the rice wine, soy sauce, and cornstarch until smooth. Add the chicken and cover; let stand 30 minutes or refrigerate up to 1 hour.

2. In a 12-inch nonstick skillet, heat the oil on medium-high. Add the green onions, garlic, and ginger; cook 3 minutes, or until the garlic is golden brown, stirring occasionally. Add the chicken and marinade; cook 3 to 5 minutes, or until the chicken is cooked through, stirring occasionally.

3. Stir in the peanuts, vinegar, and chilies; cook 2 minutes, stirring occasionally. Garnish with cilantro and serve.

SERVES 6: About 260 calories, 27g protein, 9g carbohydrates, 13g fat (2g saturated), 2g fiber, 700mg sodium.

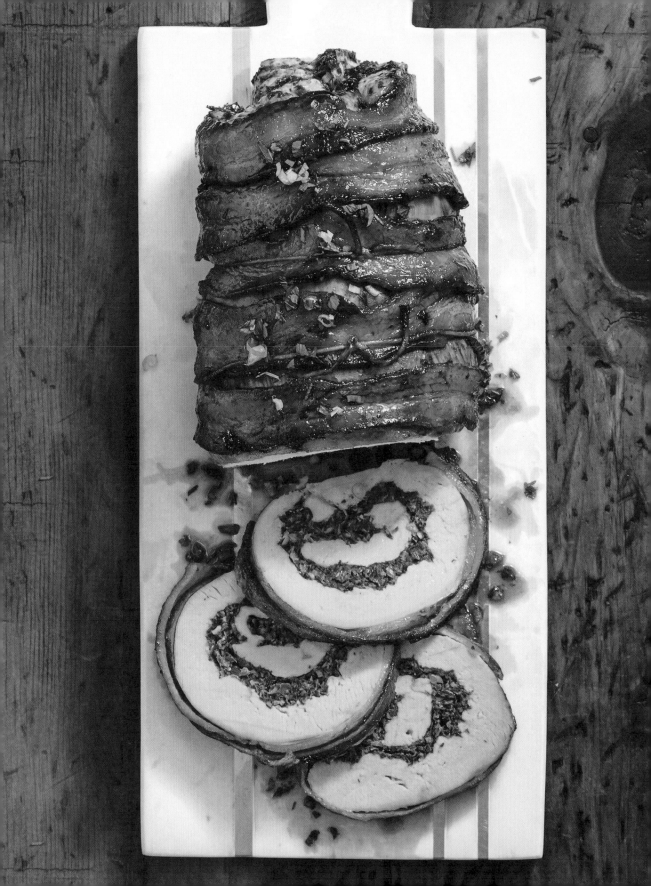

Glazed Bacon-Wrapped Turkey Breast

Whether you're entertaining and need a showstopper, or want a luscious dinner with leftovers for lunches, this bird's for you.

PREP: 20 MINUTES   TOTAL: 2 HOURS

1 boneless turkey breast (4 to 5 pounds), skin removed

¾ teaspoon kosher salt

1½ bunches green onions, sliced

2 cups packed fresh parsley

⅓ cup olive oil

4 cloves garlic

12 ounces thick-cut bacon

4 cups water

¼ cup balsamic vinegar

1. Preheat the oven to 375°F. Line a roasting pan with foil.

2. Place the turkey breast, smooth side down, on a cutting board. On the left breast, cut along the right side of the tenderloin to separate it from breast without cutting off the tenderloin; fold the tenderloin back. Repeat on the right breast, cutting along the left side of the tenderloin and folding it back. Cover the surface of the turkey with 3 large sheets of plastic wrap. With the flat side of a meat mallet or a heavy rolling pin, pound the turkey until it is about 1 inch thick all over. Discard the plastic wrap.

3. Sprinkle the surface of the turkey with the salt. In a food processor, pulse the green onions, parsley, oil, and garlic until finely chopped, stopping to stir it occasionally. Spread the herb mixture in an even layer on the turkey breast. Starting at a short side, roll up the breast tightly. Place it seam side down on the cutting board. Drape the bacon strips over the turkey roll, overlapping the slices slightly. Tuck the ends of the bacon under the turkey roll. Using 16-inch pieces of kitchen string, tie the turkey tightly at 1½-inch intervals. (At this point, the turkey may be wrapped tightly in plastic and refrigerated up to overnight.) Transfer the turkey to a rack fitted into the prepared roasting pan. Add the water to the bottom of the pan. Roast 45 minutes.

4. Brush the vinegar over turkey, return it to the oven, and roast another 45 minutes, or until the turkey is cooked through (160°F), basting it with vinegar every 15 minutes. Remove the turkey from the oven, loosely cover it with foil, and let rest 20 minutes. Cut and discard the strings before slicing and serving.

SERVES 10: About 380 calories, 54g protein, 4g carbohydrates, 15g fat (4g saturated), 1g fiber, 508mg sodium.

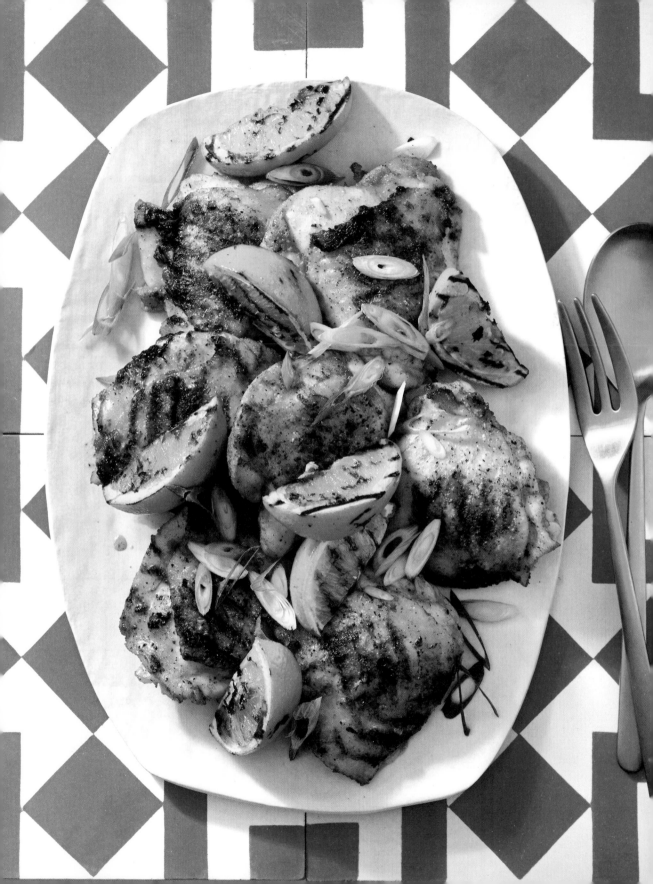

Chipotle Orange Chicken

Chipotles are smoked jalapeños and are also available canned whole in adobo sauce. If you have the canned ones, use half a chili with a spoonful of the sauce and cut the salt back to ½ teaspoon.

PREP: 5 MINUTES   TOTAL: 35 MINUTES

2 teaspoons chipotle chili powder

1 teaspoon ground cumin

1 teaspoon garlic powder

½ teaspoon onion powder

1 teaspoon kosher salt

1 teaspoon ground black pepper

4 pounds small chicken thighs, trimmed of excess skin

2 tablespoons olive oil

2 small oranges, cut into quarters

2 green onions, thinly sliced, for garnish

1. Preheat the grill on medium. In a small bowl, combine the chipotle, cumin, garlic powder, onion powder, salt, and black pepper. In a large bowl or 3-quart baking dish, toss the chicken with the oil; sprinkle it with the spice mixture, then rub the spices into the chicken to coat it evenly.

2. Grill the chicken, covered, 20 to 25 minutes, or until the chicken is cooked through (165°F), turning it once. Grill the oranges 5 to 10 minutes, or until grill marks appear. Transfer the chicken to a serving platter. Squeeze the juice from the oranges all over the chicken. Garnish with green onions and serve.

SERVES 6: About 480 calories, 42g protein, 6g carbohydrates, 31g fat (8g saturated), 1g fiber, 535mg sodium.

Cilantro-Lime Chicken

A side of simply roasted green beans would go well with this. Toss a pound of veggies with 2 tablespoons oil and add to the oven during the last 15 minutes of cooking.

PREP: 35 MINUTES   TOTAL: 1 HOUR 20 MINUTES, PLUS MARINATING

1 cup packed fresh cilantro leaves

1 cup packed fresh mint leaves

¼ cup packed fresh tarragon leaves

½ cup olive oil

⅓ cup soy sauce

¼ cup lime juice

3 tablespoons cider vinegar

5 cloves garlic

1 jalapeño chili, sliced

2 tablespoons chopped peeled fresh ginger

1 teaspoon dried oregano

1 teaspoon ground cumin

1 teaspoon kosher salt

12 assorted small chicken parts (about 3 pounds)

⅓ cup mayonnaise

1. In a food processor, puree the herbs with the oil, soy sauce, lime juice, vinegar, garlic, jalapeño, ginger, oregano, cumin, and salt until smooth. Transfer ¾ cup to small bowl; cover and refrigerate. Transfer the remaining marinade to a gallon size resealable plastic bag; add the chicken. Seal the bag, tossing to coat the chicken, and refrigerate at least 5 hours or up to overnight.

2. Preheat the oven to 375°F. Place a wire rack in a foil-lined rimmed baking sheet. Arrange the chicken on the rack, discarding the marinade in the bag; bake 30 minutes. Increase the oven temp to 450°F and roast another 15 to 20 minutes, or until the chicken is cooked through (165°F).

3. Whisk the mayonnaise into the reserved marinade. Serve the chicken with the green sauce.

SERVES 6: About 500 calories, 32g protein, 4g carbohydrates, 39g fat (8g saturated), 1g fiber, 1,140mg sodium.

Chicken Caprese

Mozzarella will up your keto ratios. With 65 percent fat and 32 percent protein and only 3 percent carbs, it's a good choice for cooking and snacking.

PREP: 15 MINUTES   TOTAL: 25 MINUTES

3 tablespoons olive oil

4 chicken breast cutlets (about 1¼ pounds)

1¼ pounds tomatoes, chopped

3 cloves garlic, sliced

½ teaspoon kosher salt

8 ounces mini fresh mozzarella balls, halved

2 tablespoons chopped fresh basil

Roasted or steamed Broccolini®, for serving

1. In a 12-inch skillet, heat the oil on medium-high; add the chicken and cook 6 minutes or until cooked through (165°F), turning once. Transfer the cutlets to plate and cover to keep warm.

2. To the skillet, add the tomatoes, garlic, and salt. Cook 3 minutes, stirring and scraping.

3. Top the chicken with the tomato sauce, mozzarella balls, and fresh basil. Serve with roasted or steamed Broccolini.

SERVES 4: About 475 calories, 45g protein, 12g carbohydrates, 28g fat (10g saturated), 4g fiber, 570mg sodium.

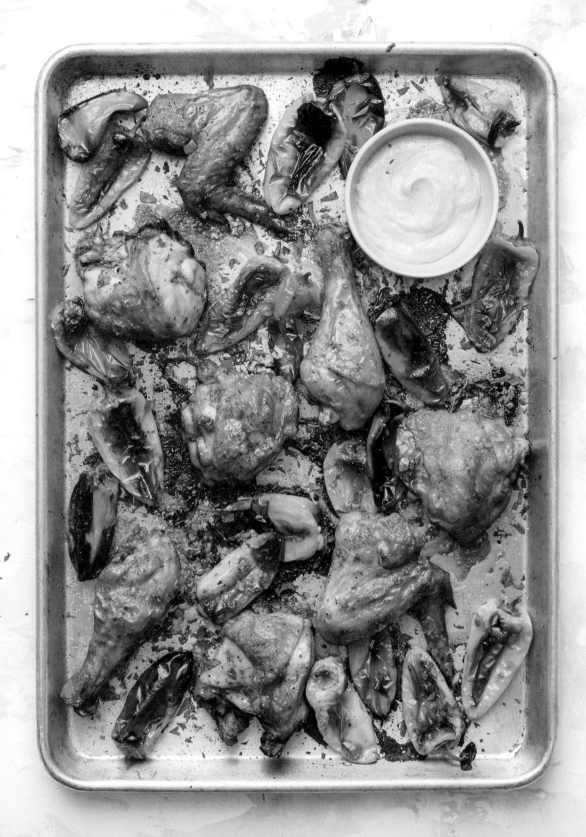

Spanish Chicken & Peppers

Mini sweet peppers add a rainbow of color and no prep time. If you don't find them in your market, use 2 bell peppers, cored, seeded, and cut into eighths.

PREP: 10 MINUTES   TOTAL: 45 MINUTES

**2½ pounds assorted small chicken parts
(cut breasts into halves)**

1 pound mini sweet peppers

1½ tablespoons olive oil

½ teaspoon kosher salt

½ teaspoon black pepper

½ cup mayonnaise

1 clove garlic, crushed with a press

¼ teaspoon smoked paprika

1. Preheat the oven to 450°F.

2. In a large bowl, toss the chicken and sweet peppers with the oil, salt, and pepper. Arrange on a rimmed baking sheet. Roast 35 minutes, or until the chicken is cooked through (165°F).

3. Meanwhile, stir together the mayonnaise, garlic, and paprika.

4. Serve the chicken and peppers with the garlic mayo.

SERVES 4: About 500 calories, 38g protein, 10g carbohydrates, 34g fat (7g saturated), 2g fiber, 595mg sodium.

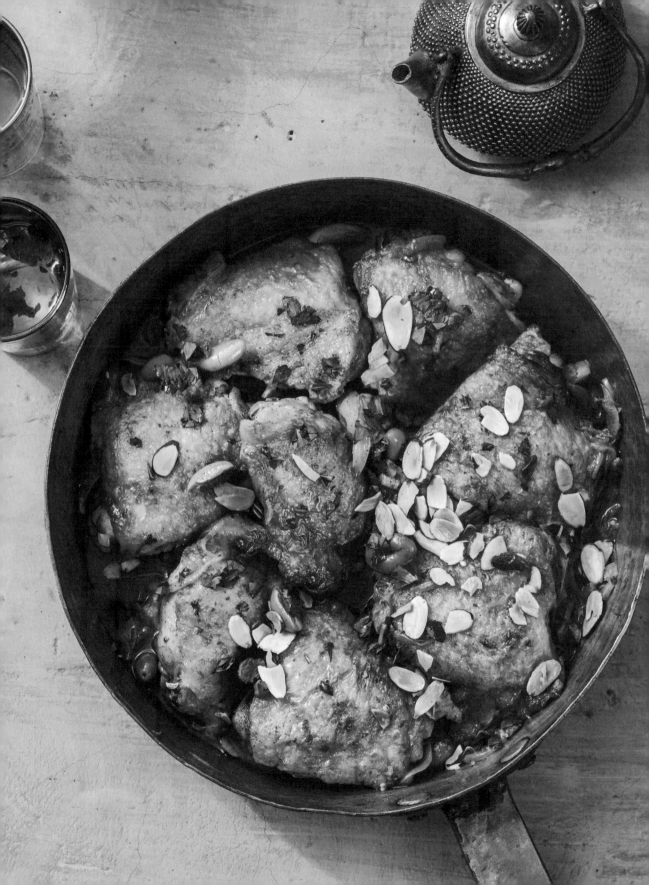

Moroccan Chicken with Preserved Lemons & Olives

This quick version of a Moroccan tagine features preserved lemons. If you don't have them, replace with a teaspoon of grated lemon zest and 2 tablespoons of juice.

PREP: 25 MINUTES   TOTAL: 50 MINUTES

2 tablespoons olive oil

8 small chicken thighs (about 2¼ pounds)

Kosher salt and ground black pepper

1 onion, thinly sliced

2 cloves garlic, finely chopped

1 teaspoon ground cumin

1 teaspoon ground cinnamon

½ teaspoon ground coriander

½ teaspoon ground ginger

1 cup low-sodium chicken broth

½ cup small pitted green olives

2 tablespoons chopped preserved lemon

¼ cup flat-leaf parsley, chopped, for garnish

Sliced toasted almonds, for garnish

1. Preheat the oven to 425°F. In a large oven-safe skillet, heat the oil on medium. Season the chicken with ½ teaspoon each salt and pepper, add to the skillet, and cook, skin side down, until golden brown and crisp, about 10 minutes. Flip and cook 1 minute more; transfer to a plate and cover to keep warm.

2. Add the onion to the skillet, cover, and cook, stirring occasionally, until tender, about 8 minutes. Uncover and stir in the garlic, cumin, cinnamon, coriander, ginger, and ½ teaspoon each salt and pepper and cook, stirring occasionally, until the onion is golden brown, 5 to 6 minutes more.

3. Stir in the broth, scraping up any browned bits. Return the chicken (along with any juices) to the skillet; stir in the olives and preserved lemon. Transfer to the oven and roast until the chicken is cooked through (165˚F), 8 to 10 minutes.

4. Sprinkle with parsley and almonds and serve.

SERVES 4: About 620 calories, 39g protein, 8g carbohydrates, 48g fat (11g saturated), 3g fiber, 987mg sodium.

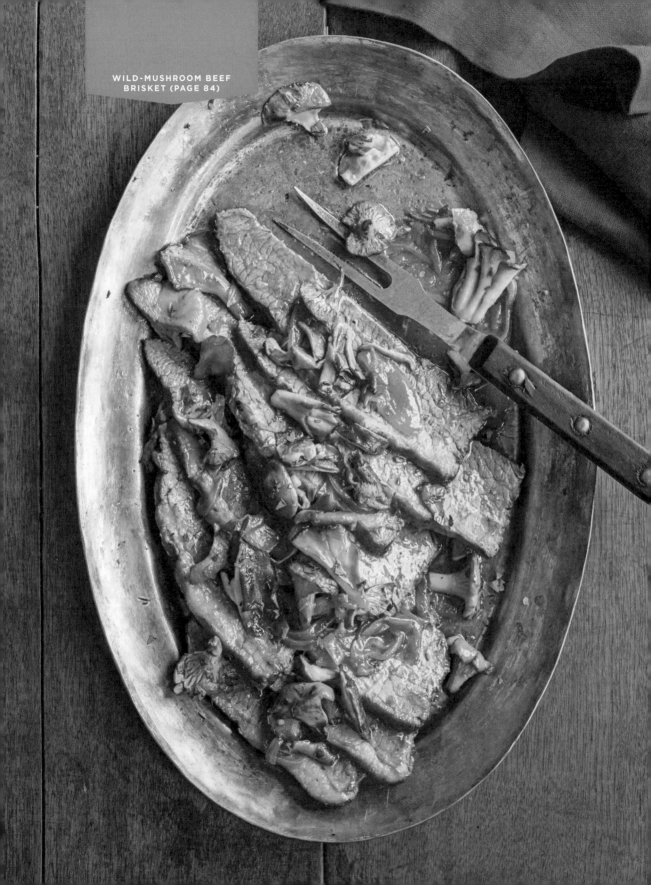

WILD-MUSHROOM BEEF
BRISKET (PAGE 84)

4 | Meat

Here are 19 meaty reasons to love keto dieting: Thick New York strip steak gets grilled and topped with a sassy green Chimichurri sauce. Brisket braised with a tumble of wild mushrooms. Slow-Cooked beef with soy paired with a fresh Tomato-Mint Salad. You get the idea. Whether you only have time to quickly sear steaks or lamb chops or you have more time and can make Two-Step Slow-Cooked Brisket, Pork Chops with Rosemary-Truffle Sauce or Sausage-Stuffed Zucchini Boats, there are delicious options that you've never seen in a diet plan before. And if you're entertaining, wow your friends with the Coffee-Rubbed Beef Tenderloin—they may just decide to try keto too!

Grilled Southwest Steak Salad ... 82

Chimichurri Strip Steak ... 83

Wild-Mushroom Beef Brisket ... 84

Coffee-Rubbed Beef Tenderloin ... 85

Soy-Braised Beef & Tomato-Mint Salad ... 87

Two-Step Slow-Cooked Brisket ... 88

Thai Steak & Pear Salad ... 91

Korean Beef Lettuce Wraps ... 93

Seared Steak with Blistered Tomatoes ... 94

Feta & Mint Mini Meatloaves ... 97

Grilled Pork with Charred Harissa Broccoli ... 99

Grilled Pork Tenderloin & Peppers ... 101

Spanish Pork Pinchos Morunos ... 102

Bacon & Eggs Over Asparagus ... 103

Grilled Pork Tenderloin with Grainy Mustard Vinaigrette ... 105

Pork Chops with Rosemary-Truffle Sauce ... 107

Sausage-Stuffed Zucchini Boats ... 109

Lebanese Kafta Kebabs ... 110

Glazed Rosemary Lamb Chops ... 111

Grilled Southwest Steak Salad

The slight bitterness of arugula stands up to the bold Southwestern flavors. If you like things really spicy add some cayenne to the steak rub.

PREP: 10 MINUTES   TOTAL: 20 MINUTES

1½ pounds skirt steak

1 teaspoon chili powder

Kosher salt

Ground black pepper

1½ pounds plum tomatoes, chopped

2 green onions, sliced

1 jalapeño chili, sliced

2 tablespoons fresh lime juice

1 cup cilantro, tough stems removed

6 cups baby arugula

1. Preheat the broiler or grill on medium-high. Season the skirt steak with chili powder and ½ teaspoon each salt and black pepper. Broil or grill to the desired doneness, 3 to 4 minutes per side for medium-rare. Let rest for 5 minutes before slicing against the grain.

2. In a large bowl, toss the plum tomatoes, green onions, jalapeño, lime juice, and salt and pepper to taste. Toss with the cilantro and arugula; fold in the sliced steak before serving.

SERVES 4: About 340 calories, 41g protein, 9g carbohydrates, 16.5g fat (5.5g saturated), 3g fiber, 595mg sodium.

Chimichurri Strip Steak

This Argentine herb sauce is a favorite for beef. We think
it would make any meat or fish more delicious.

PREP: 10 MINUTES   TOTAL: 25 MINUTES

1 cup packed fresh parsley

1 cup packed fresh cilantro

1 clove garlic

3 tablespoons extra-virgin olive oil

2 tablespoons sherry vinegar

¼ teaspoon dried oregano

¼ teaspoon crushed red pepper

Kosher salt and ground black pepper

4 New York beef strip steaks (2½ pounds),
   each 1 inch thick

Grilled Plum Tomatoes (recipe at right;
   optional)

1. Preheat the grill on medium-high. Fit a wire
rack into a rimmed baking sheet.

2. Prepare the chimichurri: In a food processor,
pulse the parsley, cilantro, and garlic until finely
chopped. Add the oil, vinegar, oregano, red
pepper, and ⅛ teaspoon each salt and black
pepper; pulse to blend.

3. Pat the steaks dry. Season with ½ teaspoon
each salt and black pepper. Grill, turning
occasionally, to the desired doneness, 7 to 8
minutes for medium-rare (135°F). Transfer to the
wire rack. Let stand 5 minutes.

4. Stir the meat juices into the chimichurri. Slice
the steak; serve with the sauce and, if desired,
grilled tomatoes.

SERVES 6 (STEAK AND SAUCE ONLY):
About 445 calories, 38g protein, 1g
carbohydrates, 31g fat (10g saturated), 1g
fiber, 285mg sodium.

Grilled Plum Tomatoes

Halve **6 medium plum tomatoes** lengthwise.
Brush the cut sides lightly with **1 tablespoon
olive oil** and sprinkle with **¼ teaspoon each
kosher salt and ground black pepper**. Grill until
lightly charred, 3 to 5 minutes per side. Serves 6.

SERVES 6: About 30 calories, 1g protein,
2g carbohydrates, 2g fat (0g saturated),
1g fiber, 83mg sodium.

Wild-Mushroom Beef Brisket

Fresh and dried mushrooms give this brisket rich flavor. Serve it with steamed cauliflower rice to catch the juices. See photo on page 80.

PREP: 30 MINUTES   TOTAL: 3 HOURS 25 MINUTES

1 ounce dried porcini mushrooms

3 cups boiling water

7 tablespoons vegetable oil, divided

1 beef brisket (4 pounds), trimmed

Kosher salt

1 teaspoon ground black pepper

2 medium onions, finely chopped

3 tablespoons balsamic vinegar

2 cups beef broth

8 sprigs fresh thyme, tied together

1 cup water

1 pound mixed wild mushrooms, sliced

2 tablespoons chopped fresh flat-leaf parsley

1. In a medium bowl, combine the dried porcinis and boiling water. Let soak 20 minutes. With a spoon, remove the porcinis from the water; coarsely chop. Strain the soaking liquid through a fine-mesh sieve; reserve the liquid and discard any sandy solids.

2. Preheat the oven to 325°F. In large, wide-bottomed Dutch oven or oven-safe saucepot, heat 3 tablespoons of the oil on medium-high until hot. Season the brisket all over with 1 teaspoon salt and the pepper. Add the brisket to the pot; cook 6 to 7 minutes, or until browned on both sides, turning once. Transfer the brisket to a large plate.

3. To the same pot, add the onions and 1 teaspoon salt. Cook 3 to 5 minutes, or until browned, stirring frequently. Add the vinegar. Cook 1 minute or until reduced, scraping up any browned bits with wooden spoon.

4. To the pot, add the chopped porcinis, reserved soaking liquid, broth, thyme, brisket, and water. Heat to boiling on high. Cover and place in the oven. Cook 3 to 3½ hours, or until the brisket is very tender. Remove and discard the thyme. Skim and discard any fat.

5. Meanwhile, in a 12-inch skillet, heat the remaining 4 tablespoons oil on medium-high. Add the sliced mushrooms and 1 teaspoon salt. Cook 15 minutes, or until browned and tender, stirring occasionally. Remove from the heat and add the parsley, tossing to combine. To serve, thinly slice the brisket and return it to the pot, pouring the cooking liquid over meat, and topping it with the sautéed mushrooms.

SERVES 10: About 390 calories, 42g protein, 10g carbohydrates, 20g fat (5g saturated), 2g fiber, 655 mg sodium.

Coffee-Rubbed Beef Tenderloin

The tenderest cut gets spiced with smoky paprika and cayenne along with the coffee to give it smokehouse flavor. Serve any leftovers in salads or in lettuce cups with the sweet pepper sauce.

PREP: 15 MINUTES   TOTAL: 1 HOUR, PLUS MARINATING

1 trimmed beef tenderloin
  (about 4 pounds), tied

1 tablespoon vegetable oil

3 tablespoons ground coffee

1 teaspoon cayenne pepper

2 teaspoons smoked paprika

2 teaspoons garlic powder

2 teaspoons kosher salt

1 teaspoon ground black pepper

4 cups water

Sweet Pepper Sauce (recipe at right)

1. Place the tenderloin on a very large sheet of plastic wrap and brush it with the oil. In medium bowl, combine the coffee, cayenne, paprika, garlic powder, salt, and black pepper; rub the mixture all over the beef, patting it to adhere. Wrap the beef tightly in plastic and refrigerate at least 1 hour or up to 4 hours.

2. Preheat the oven to 450°F. Remove the beef from the plastic and place it on a rack set in a roasting pan. Pour the water into the bottom of the pan. Roast 45 to 55 minutes, or to the desired doneness (135°F for medium-rare). Let stand at least 10 minutes before serving. Serve the beef thinly sliced with the sauce.

SERVES 12 (with 2 tablespoons sauce):
310 calories, 32g protein, 6g carbohydrates, 17g fat (5g saturated), 2g fiber, 650mg sodium.

Sweet Pepper Sauce

In a food processor, pulse **1½ cups roasted red peppers, 2 tablespoons tomato paste, 1 cup blanched sliced almonds, 1 cup canola or vegetable oil, 2 tablespoons sherry vinegar, 1 clove garlic,** and **1 teaspoon kosher salt** until smooth. Makes 2 cups.

EACH 2-TABLESPOON SERVING: About 85 calories, 0g protein, 3g carbohydrates, 8g fat (0g saturated), 1g fiber, 120mg sodium.

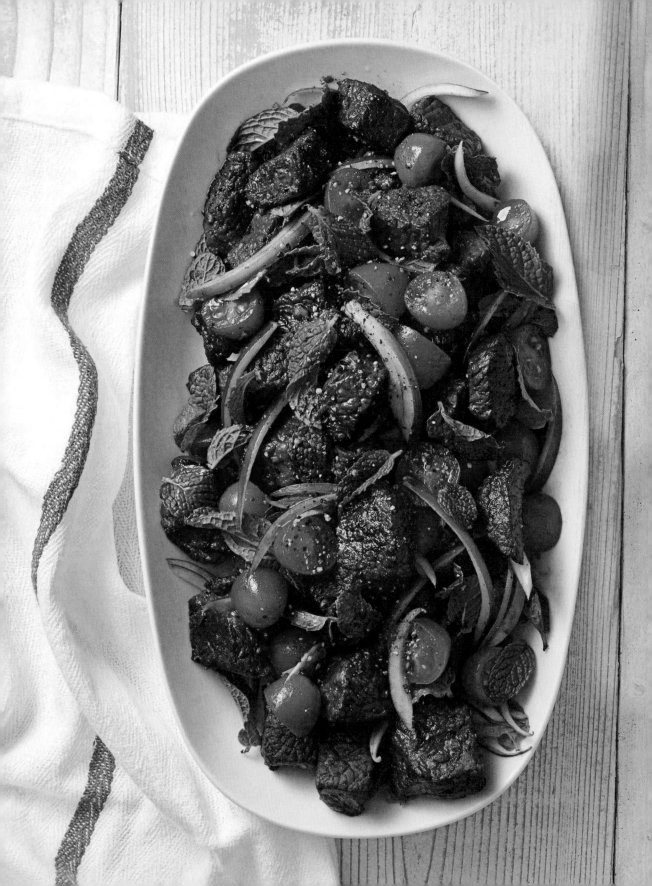

Soy-Braised Beef & Tomato-Mint Salad

This slow-cooker braise is a riff on Vietnamese shaking beef.
Serve with a pile of lettuce leaves for wrapping if you like.

PREP: 15 MINUTES   TOTAL: 6 HOURS 15 MINUTES

3 pounds beef brisket, trimmed of excess fat and cut into 1-inch chunks

5 cloves garlic, chopped

¼ cup rice vinegar

¼ cup soy sauce

3 tablespoons fish sauce

½ teaspoon ground black pepper

1 pint grape tomatoes, halved

1 small red onion, thinly sliced

½ cup mint leaves

Liquid stevia (optional)

In a 7- to 8-quart slow-cooker bowl, combine the beef brisket, garlic, rice vinegar, soy sauce, fish sauce, and pepper. Cook on Low 6 to 8 hours, or until tender; toss with the grape tomatoes, red onion, and mint leaves. Add a few drops stevia, if desired, and serve.

SERVES 6: About 290 calories, 42g protein, 9g carbohydrates, 10g fat (4g saturated), 2g fiber, 510mg sodium

Two-Step Slow-Cooked Brisket

The second step, roasting onions until caramelized
and sweet elevates this simple brisket.

1 beef brisket (about 4 pounds), trimmed

Kosher salt

¾ teaspoon ground black pepper

1 can (14 ounces) crushed tomatoes

3 cloves garlic, crushed with a press

1 medium red onion, sliced

1 medium yellow onion, sliced

1 tablespoon olive oil

Finely chopped fresh parsley, for topping

1. Season the brisket with ¾ teaspoon salt and
the pepper; place it in a large slow-cooker bowl
along with crushed tomatoes and garlic. Cover
and cook on Low 10 hours, or until very tender.

2. About 25 minutes before the meat is ready,
preheat the oven to 425°F. On a large rimmed
baking sheet, toss the red and yellow onions with
the oil and ¼ teaspoon salt. Roast 20 minutes, or
until browned. To serve, top the brisket with the
roasted onions and finely chopped parsley.

SERVES 6: About 300 calories, 35g protein,
9g carbohydrates, 14g fat (4g saturated),
2g fiber, 590mg sodium.

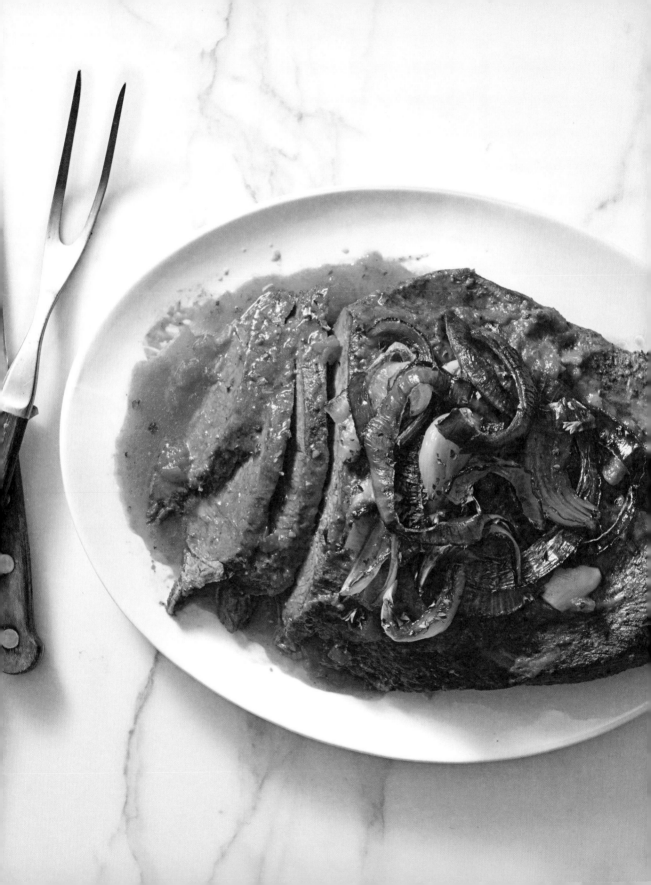

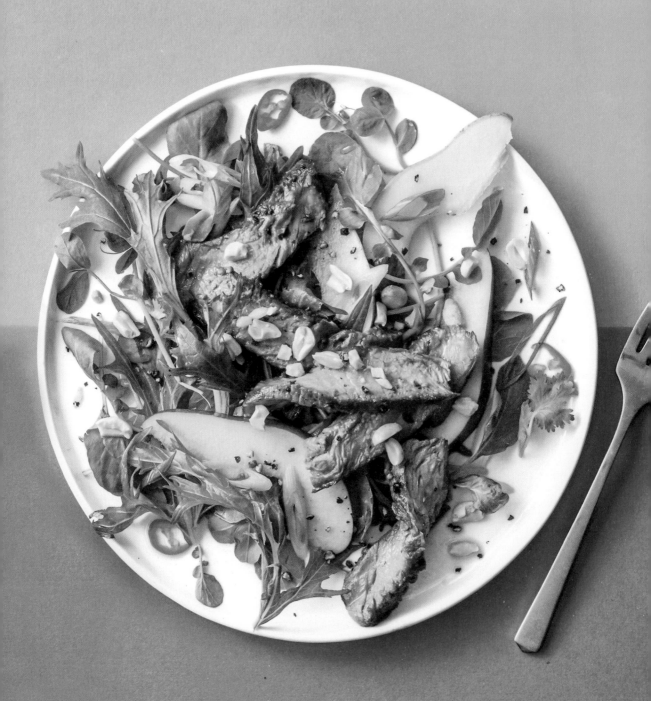

Thai Steak & Pear Salad

A small amount of sweet pear (and other fruit) is okay for keto and is the perfect balance to the salty tang of lime and fish sauce. You could also make this with grilled chicken or shrimp.

PREP: 15 MINUTES   TOTAL: 20 MINUTES

1¼ pounds strip steak, trimmed

½ teaspoon kosher salt

½ teaspoon ground black pepper

4 tablespoons fresh lime juice

1 tablespoon fish sauce

1 teaspoon water

1 small Bartlett pear, thinly sliced

2 green onions, thinly sliced

1 small red hot chili pepper, thinly sliced

5 ounces mixed greens

1 cup cilantro, chopped

Chopped peanuts, for serving
(optional)

1. Heat a medium cast-iron skillet on medium-high. Season the strip steak with salt and black pepper and cook to the desired doneness, 3 to 4 minutes per side for medium-rare. Transfer the meat to a cutting board; let rest 5 minutes before slicing.

2. Meanwhile, in a large bowl, combine the lime juice, fish sauce, and water. Add the pear, green onions, and red chili and toss to combine. Fold in the mixed greens and cilantro.

3. Serve the salad with the steak and sprinkle with chopped peanuts, if desired.

SERVES 4: About 245 calories, 31g protein, 11g carbohydrates, 8.5g fat (3.5g saturated), 2g fiber, 615mg sodium.

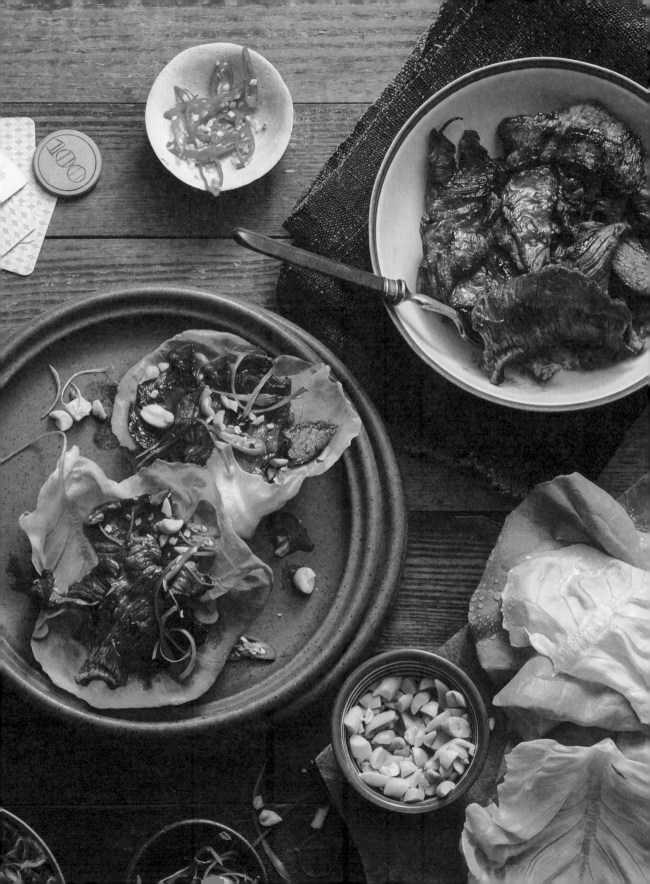

Korean Beef Lettuce Wraps

Fresh ginger adds flavor and tenderizes the meat.
The key to slicing it thinly is the freezing time.

TOTAL: 20 MINUTES, PLUS FREEZING AND MARINATING

¼ cup water

1 clove garlic, grated

2 tablespoons low-sodium soy sauce

½ teaspoon crushed red pepper

1 tablespoon grated peeled fresh ginger

1 tablespoon toasted sesame oil

1 pound sirloin, strip steak, or boneless
 short rib, frozen until just solid
 (45 to 60 minutes)

2 tablespoons canola oil, divided

Kosher salt

Lettuce leaves, sliced green onions, sliced
 red chilies, and chopped peanuts,
 for serving (optional)

1. In a medium bowl, combine the water, garlic, soy sauce, crushed red pepper, ginger, and sesame oil. Thinly slice the frozen meat, add to the marinade, and toss to coat. Let marinate at room temperature 30 minutes or cover and refrigerate up to 3 hours. Remove from refrigerator 30 minutes before cooking.

2. Heat a large stainless-steel skillet on medium-high. Add 1 tablespoon of the oil. Transfer half the beef mixture to the skillet, arrange in even layer, season with ¼ teaspoon salt, and cook without moving until lightly browned, about 1 minute. Toss the beef and continue to cook until just cooked through and crisp at the edges, about 2 more minutes. Transfer to a plate and keep warm. Repeat with the remaining tablespoon oil and beef.

3. Serve immediately with lettuce leaves, green onions, chilies, and peanuts, if desired.

SERVES 6 (steak only): About 190 calories, 15g protein, 1g carbohydrates, 13.5g fat (4.5g saturated), 0g fiber, 245mg sodium.

Seared Steak with Blistered Tomatoes

Using high heat to sear and blister veggies amps their flavors. If you can't find cherry tomatoes on the vine, use a pint of grape tomatoes. See photo on page 2.

PREP: 5 MINUTES   TOTAL: 20 MINUTES

2 strip steaks (about 1½ pounds),
    each 1½ inches thick

Kosher salt and ground black pepper

4 tablespoons olive oil, divided

6 cloves garlic, unpeeled

2 bunches cherry tomatoes on the vine
    (about 1½ pounds)

2 sprigs fresh rosemary

2 tablespoons white wine vinegar

¼ small red onion, finely chopped

3 tablespoons crumbled blue cheese
    (about 1 ounce)

Arugula, for serving

1. Preheat the oven to 450°F. Heat a large cast-iron skillet on medium-high. Season the steaks with ¼ teaspoon each salt and pepper. Add 1 teaspoon of the oil to the skillet, then add the steaks and garlic and cook until the steaks are browned, 3 minutes per side.

2. Add the tomatoes on the vine and rosemary to the skillet, drizzle with 2 teaspoons of the oil, and season with salt and pepper. Transfer the skillet to the oven and roast until the steak is at the desired degree of doneness, 3 to 4 minutes for medium-rare, and the tomatoes begin to slightly break down. Transfer the steaks to a cutting board and let rest at least 5 minutes before serving. Transfer the tomatoes and garlic to a platter; squeeze the garlic cloves from their skins.

3. In a small bowl, combine the vinegar, the remaining 3 tablespoons oil, and ¼ teaspoon each salt and pepper; stir in the onion and fold in the blue cheese. Serve the steak, tomatoes, garlic, and the arugula drizzled with vinaigrette.

SERVES 4: About 445 calories, 39g protein, 9g carbohydrates, 28g fat (8.5g saturated), 2g fiber, 455mg sodium.

> **TIP**
>
> To make the best-ever pan sauce, as soon as your meat is done cooking, transfer it to a plate. Add wine or broth to the hot skillet. Use a wooden spoon to stir everything together, scraping up the brown bits left in the pan. Whisk in heavy cream and mustard or another condiment, and voilà!

Roasting Vegetables

• Avoid overcrowding. Space food out, or it will steam instead of brown. Use a large rimmed baking sheet or two smaller ones, switching them between racks halfway through.

• Turn up the heat. The magic temp to cook quickly and maximize browning is 450°F.

VEGETABLES	HOW TO CUT	ROASTING TIME AT 450°F	GARNISH & SERVING
Asparagus	Trimmed	10 to 15 minutes	Garnish with 1 teaspoon freshly grated lemon
Broccoli	Trim and peel stem, split florets into 1½-inch-wide pieces	10 to 15 minutes	Sprinkle with 1 tablespoon grated Cheddar cheese
Brussels Sprouts	Trim and halve through stem end	15 to 20 minutes	Season with salt and pepper, serve immediately
Cauliflower	1½-inch florets	20 to 30 minutes	Sprinkle with 2 tablespoons chopped fresh parsley
Eggplant	½-inch-thick slices	20 to 25 minutes	Drizzle with 1 tablespoon extra-virgin olive oil
Fennel	Trim and cut into 12 wedges	35 to 40 minutes	Garnish with ½ teaspoon freshly grated orange peel
Green Beans	Trim ends	20 to 30 minutes	Toss with 2 tablespoons each lemon juice and chopped fresh dill
Onions	Cut into wedges	20 to 30 minutes	Remove onions from oven and brush with mixture of 1 tablespoon brown sugar, 1 teaspoon apple cider vinegar. Return to oven and roast for 5 more minutes
Sweet Peppers	1-inch-wide strips	30 minutes	Garnish with 3 basil leaves, thinly sliced
Turnips	Peel and cut into 6 wedges	45 to 50 minutes	Garnish with 1 tablespoon chopped fresh mint
Zucchini	Trim and cut in half crosswise then each half quartered	15 to 20 minutes	Garnish with 1 tablespoon freshly grated Parmesan

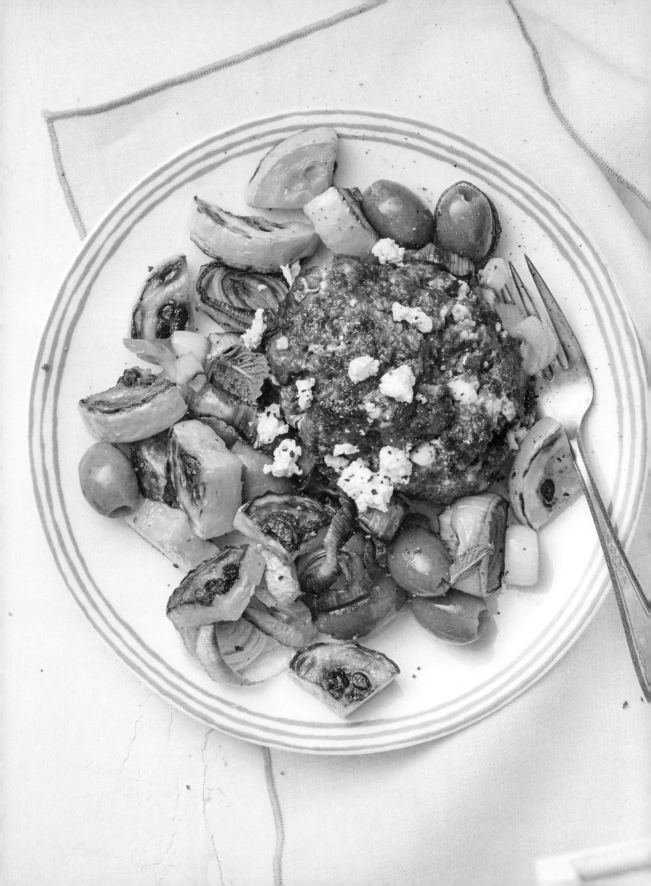

Feta & Mint Mini Meatloaves

The briny flavors of this Greek meatloaf need a fatty meat like chuck for balance. If you like lamb, it would also be an excellent choice.

PREP: 15 MINUTES   TOTAL: 30 MINUTES

1¼ pounds ground beef chuck

½ cup crumbled feta cheese

½ cup fresh mint, finely chopped

Kosher salt

1 large leek, sliced

3 medium yellow squash, chopped

1 cup pitted green olives

1 tablespoon olive oil

1. Preheat the oven to 450°F. In a bowl, combine the beef chuck, feta, mint, and ¼ teaspoon salt. Divide the mixture into fourths and form 4 mini loaves, placing them on a rimmed baking sheet.

2. In a separate bowl, toss the leek, squash, and olives with the oil and ⅛ teaspoon salt; arrange the vegetables around the loaves on the baking sheet.

3. Roast 15 to 20 minutes, or until the meatloaves are cooked through (165°F).

4. Serve the meatloaves with the vegetables.

SERVES 4: About 415 calories, 30g protein, 12g carbohydrates, 28g fat (10g saturated), 4g fiber, 935mg sodium.

TIP

In our tests, dark-colored pans held too much heat and overbrowned foods. Go light—even if you choose a baking sheet with a nonstick finish.

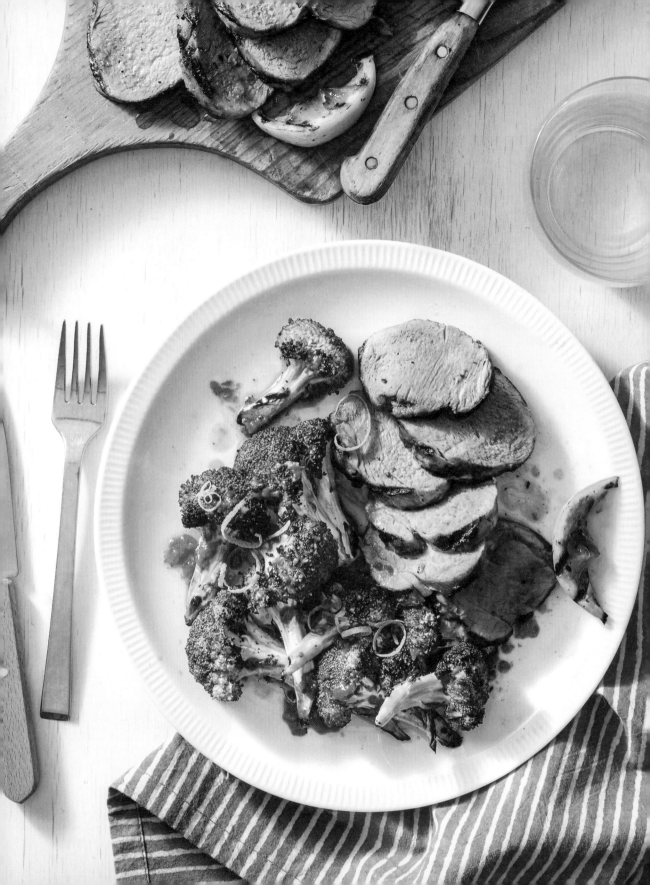

Grilled Pork with Charred Harissa Broccoli

Pork tenderloin is a lean protein powerhouse and a perfect canvas for multiple flavors. Look for harissa, a spicy North African condiment in your market.

PREP: 10 MINUTES   TOTAL: 30 MINUTES

2 lemons

1½ pounds pork tenderloin

3 tablespoons plus 1 teaspoon olive oil, divided

½ teaspoon kosher salt

Ground black pepper

1 large head broccoli (about 1¼ pounds), trimmed and cut into large florets

2 tablespoons harissa

1. Preheat the grill on medium-high. Finely grate the zest of 1 lemon and set it aside, then cut both lemons in half. Brush the pork with 1 teaspoon of the oil and season it with the salt and pepper. Grill the pork, turning it occasionally, until it reaches 140°F on an instant-read thermometer, 18 to 20 minutes. Transfer the pork to a cutting board and let rest at least 5 minutes.

2. Meanwhile, coat the broccoli with 1 tablespoon of the oil and grill it alongside the pork, turning often, until just tender and charred, 8 to 10 minutes. Grill the lemons until charred, 1 to 2 minutes.

3. In a small bowl, mix the harissa with the remaining 2 tablespoons oil and toss it with the grilled broccoli; sprinkle the lemon zest on top.

4. Squeeze two grilled lemon halves over the pork, then slice it. Serve with broccoli and remaining grilled lemon, cut into wedges.

SERVES 4: About 330 calories, 38g protein, 8g carbohydrates, 16.5g fat (3.5g saturated), 3g fiber, 385mg sodium.

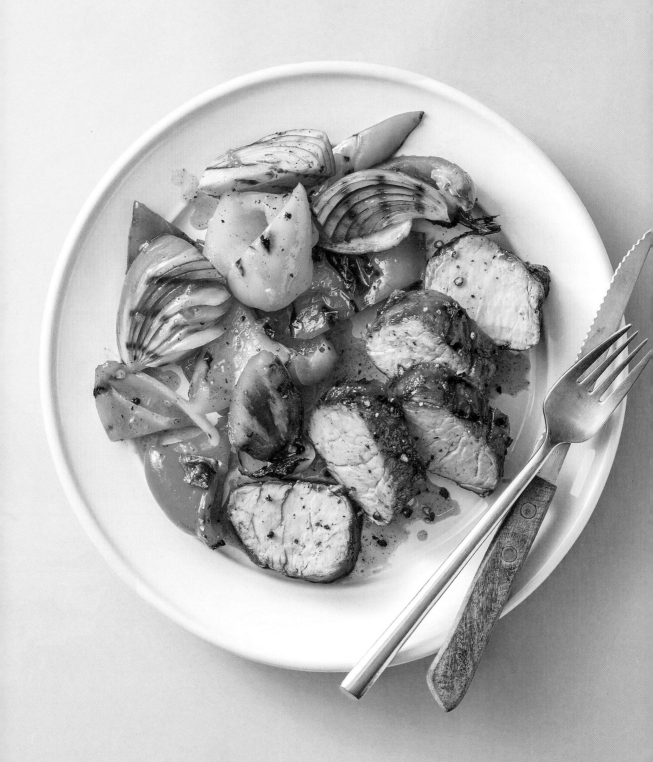

Grilled Pork Tenderloin & Peppers

Sweet bell peppers are an excellent source of Vitamin C. Did you know that one pepper gives you 250 percent of your recommended daily value?

PREP: 10 MINUTES   TOTAL: 25 MINUTES

4 peppers (red, yellow, orange, or a combination), quartered

1 red onion, cut into ½-inch wedges

1 tablespoon olive oil

Kosher salt and ground black pepper

2 small pork tenderloins (about ¾ pound each)

2 tablespoons balsamic vinegar

1. Preheat a grill on medium-high. In a bowl, toss the peppers and red onion with the oil and season with salt and black pepper to taste.

2. Season the pork tenderloins with ¼ teaspoon each salt and black pepper. Cover and grill the vegetables and pork, turning occasionally, until the vegetables are tender, 8 to 10 minutes. Transfer the vegetables to a cutting board.

3. Continue grilling the pork, basting it with the balsamic, until cooked through (145°F), 3 to 6 minutes. Let rest 5 minutes before slicing. Coarsely chop the peppers and serve with onion and pork.

SERVES 4: About 275 calories, 36g protein, 12g carbohydrates, 9g fat (2g saturated), 3g fiber, 231mg sodium.

Spanish Pork Pinchos Morunos

Serve these savory skewers with Tapas Salad
(page 128) for a total immersion Spanish dinner.

TOTAL: 25 MINUTES, PLUS MARINATING

2 tablespoons olive oil

2 tablespoons sherry vinegar

2 large cloves garlic, crushed with a press

¼ cup flat-leaf parsley, finely chopped

2 tablespoons fresh thyme leaves, chopped

2 teaspoons smoked paprika

1 teaspoon dried oregano

½ teaspoon ground cumin

½ teaspoon ground coriander

½ teaspoon kosher salt

½ teaspoon ground black pepper

1½ pounds pork tenderloin, cut into 1-inch cubes

1. In a large bowl, combine the oil, vinegar, garlic, parsley, thyme, spices, salt, and pepper. Toss the pork cubes with the marinade; cover and refrigerate at least 1 hour or up to overnight.

2. Preheat a grill on medium-high. Thread the pork onto skewers; grill, turning occasionally, until charred and just cooked through, 6 to 8 minutes.

SERVES 4: About 285 calories, 37g protein, 1g carbohydrates, 13.5g fat (4g saturated), 0g fiber, 200mg sodium.

Bacon & Eggs Over Asparagus

Bacon and eggs get a springtime boost with asparagus.
To prevent breaking the yolks, crack each egg, one at a time,
into a small cup or bowl, then pour onto the asparagus.

PREP: 8 MINUTES   **TOTAL: 30 MINUTES**

8 slices bacon

1 pound asparagus spears, trimmed

½ teaspoon fresh thyme leaves, chopped

Ground black pepper

8 large eggs

⅛ teaspoon kosher salt

3 tablespoons packed fresh flat-leaf parsley leaves, chopped

1 tablespoon fresh dill, chopped

1. Preheat the oven to 475°F. In an 18 × 12-inch jelly-roll pan, arrange the bacon slices in single layer, spacing them ¼ inch apart. Roast 8 to 9 minutes, or until browned and crisp. Transfer to a paper-towel-lined plate; set aside. Drain and discard the excess bacon fat, leaving a thin film of fat in the pan.

2. Add the asparagus to the pan in a single layer. Roll them in the fat until evenly coated. Arrange them in a tight single layer, with the bottoms of the spears touching one long side of pan. Sprinkle the thyme and ¼ teaspoon pepper on the asparagus. Roast 8 to 10 minutes, or until the asparagus spears are tender and browned.

3. Carefully crack eggs, without breaking the yolks, directly onto the asparagus spears, spacing them 1 inch apart and staggering them if necessary. Carefully return the pan to the oven. Roast 5 to 6 minutes, or until the whites are just set and the yolks are still runny. Sprinkle the salt and ⅛ teaspoon pepper on the eggs. Return the bacon to the pan; sprinkle the eggs and asparagus with the parsley and dill. To serve, use wide spatula to transfer the asparagus and eggs to serving plates.

SERVES 4: About 245 calories, 20g protein, 4g carbohydrates, 16g fat (5g saturated), 1g fiber, 486mg sodium.

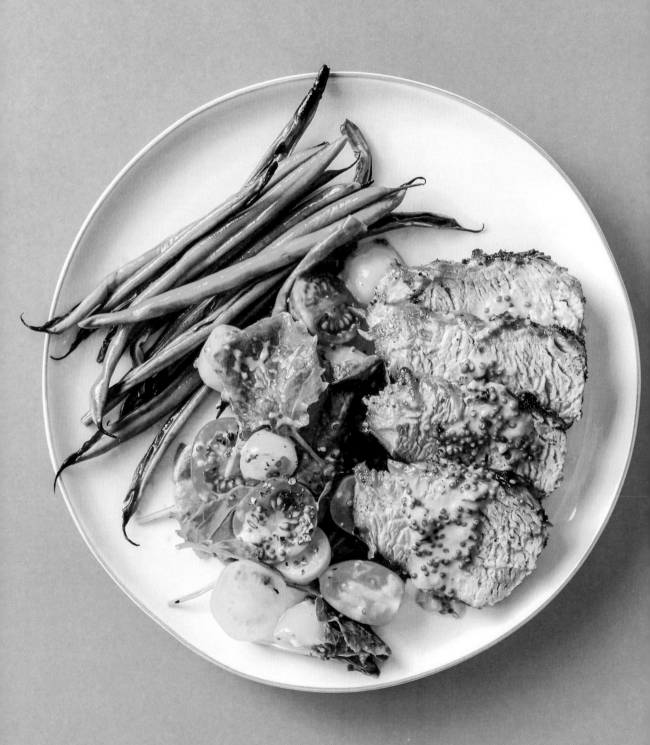

Grilled Pork Tenderloin with Grainy Mustard Vinaigrette

Not grilling tonight? Preheat the oven to 450°F
and roast your beans and pork 18 to 20 minutes.

PREP: 5 MINUTES   TOTAL: 35 MINUTES

12 ounces green beans, trimmed

Olive oil

Kosher salt

1 pork tenderloin (1¼ pounds)

½ teaspoon ground black pepper

3 tablespoons no-salt-added grainy mustard

2 tablespoons red wine vinegar

1 small shallot, finely chopped

1 teaspoon mayonnaise

6 cups baby kale

1 pint grape tomatoes, halved lengthwise

1. Preheat a grill on medium. In a bowl, toss the green beans with 1 teaspoon oil and ¼ teaspoon salt; arrange the beans on one half of a large sheet of heavy-duty foil. Fold the foil over; crimp to seal tightly. Cover and grill for 20 minutes.

2. Meanwhile, brush the pork tenderloin with 2 teaspoons oil; season with ½ teaspoon salt and the pepper. Cover and grill, turning occasionally, until cooked through (145°F), 18 to 20 minutes. Let rest 5 minutes; slice.

3. To make the vinaigrette, whisk together the grainy mustard, vinegar, shallot, 1 tablespoon oil, mayonnaise, and ¼ teaspoon salt.

4. Toss the baby kale and grape tomatoes with half of the vinaigrette. Serve with the grilled beans, pork, and the remaining vinaigrette.

SERVES 4: About 290 calories, 32g protein, 11g carbohydrates, 13g fat (3g saturated), 5g fiber, 595mg sodium.

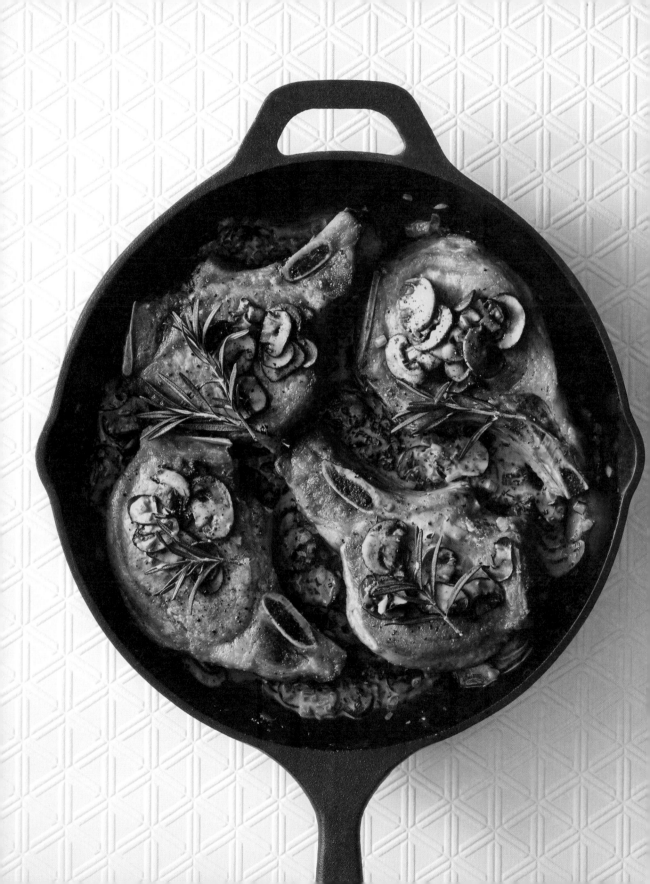

Pork Chops with Rosemary-Truffle Sauce

We think truffle butter can make anything taste good. Here thick pork chops get seared and finished with a creamy mushroom-shallot sauce—delicious.

PREP: 15 MINUTES   TOTAL: 30 MINUTES

2 tablespoons olive oil

4 bone-in pork chops, each about 1 inch thick

Kosher salt

½ teaspoon ground black pepper

3 medium shallots, chopped

12 ounces cremini mushrooms, thinly sliced

½ teaspoon chopped fresh rosemary

⅔ cup half-and-half

2 tablespoons truffle butter

1. In a 12-inch skillet, heat the oil on medium-high until hot but not smoking. Season the pork chops all over with ½ teaspoon salt and the pepper. Cook the pork chops 6 minutes, or until browned on both sides, turning them over once; transfer to a large plate and cover to keep warm. Reduce the heat to medium and pour off any excess fat in skillet. To the skillet, add the shallots, mushrooms, rosemary, and ⅛ teaspoon salt. Cook 5 minutes, stirring occasionally.

2. Stir in the half-and-half and truffle butter. Nestle the pork chops in the sauce. Simmer 4 to 6 minutes, or until the pork is cooked through (145°F).

SERVES 4: About 400 calories, 33g protein, 9g carbohydrates, 25g fat (10 g saturated), 1g fiber, 400mg sodium.

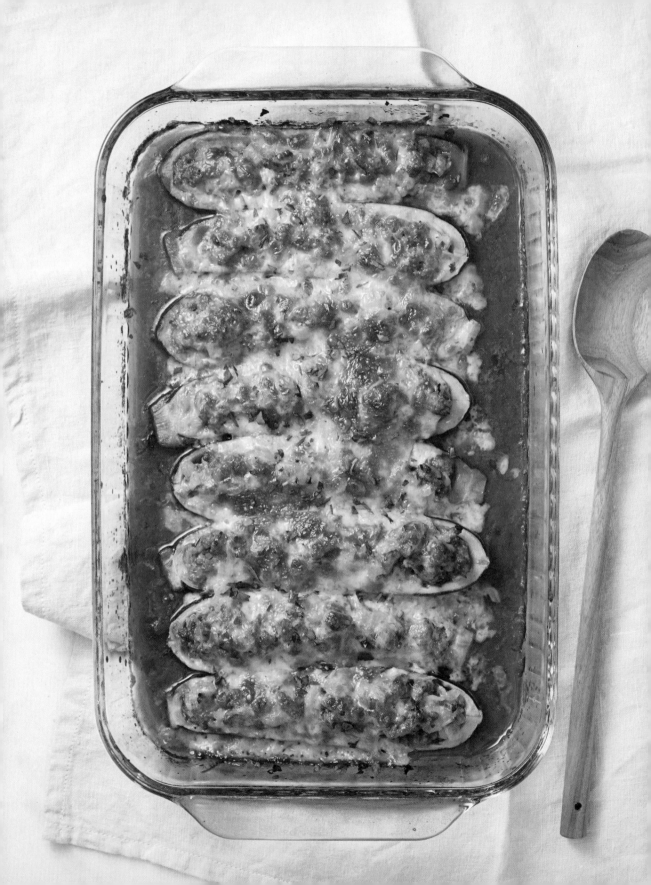

Sausage-Stuffed Zucchini Boats

This dish will be a hit with your whole family. Serve it
with Lemony Brussels Sprouts Salad (page 131).

PREP: 20 MINUTES   TOTAL: 55 MINUTES

4 small zucchini

2 teaspoons olive oil

1 small onion, chopped

2 links sweet Italian sausage,
    casing removed

¼ teaspoon kosher salt

1¼ cups no-sugar-added marinara sauce

1 cup shredded mozzarella

Chopped parsley, for garnish

1. Preheat the oven to 450°F.

2. Cut each zucchini in half lengthwise; scoop
out and chop the flesh, leaving a ¼-inch shell.

3. In a 10-inch skillet, heat the oil on medium-
high. Add the chopped zucchini, onion, Italian
sausage, and salt. Cook 8 minutes, breaking up
the sausage with the back of a spoon.

4. In a 3-quart baking dish, spread the marinara
sauce evenly on the bottom; arrange the
zucchini shells on top, cut sides up. Spoon the
sausage mixture evenly into the shells. Top with
shredded mozzarella. Cover with foil; bake 30
minutes. Uncover and bake 5 more minutes.
Garnish with chopped parsley and serve.

SERVES 4: About 325 calories, 16g protein,
15g carbohydrates, 23g fat (9g saturated),
3g fiber, 925mg sodium.

Lebanese Kafta Kebabs

Serve these spiced kebabs with Feta-Dill Greek Caesar (page 126). If you like, you can make the meat mixture the night before, so the spices will meld with the meat.

(page 126)

TOTAL: 25 MINUTES

8 ounces ground lamb

8 ounces ground beef

½ small onion, grated

2 large cloves garlic, crushed with a press

⅓ cup mint, finely chopped

½ cup flat-leaf parsley, finely chopped

2 teaspoons ground cumin

2 teaspoons ground coriander

1 teaspoon ground sumac

½ teaspoon ground allspice

½ teaspoon kosher salt

½ teaspoon ground black pepper

1. Preheat a grill or grill pan on medium-high. In a medium bowl, combine all the ingredients until well blended. Shape into 1½-inch balls and thread about 3 onto each skewer.

2. Grill the skewers, turning occasionally, until cooked through, 6 to 8 minutes.

SERVES 4: About 230 calories, 21g protein, 4g carbohydrates, 14.5g fat (5.5g saturated), 2g fiber, 335mg sodium.

Glazed Rosemary Lamb Chops

If you want to use rack of lamb, cut it into 2 chop portions.
Serve with Asparagus with Eggs Mimosa (page 135).

Serve with Asparagus with Eggs Mimosa (page 135).

PREP: 10 MINUTES   TOTAL: 20 MINUTES

8 lamb loin chops (4 ounces each),
   each 1 inch thick

1 large clove garlic, cut in half

2 teaspoons chopped fresh rosemary,
   or ½ teaspoon dried rosemary, crumbled

¼ teaspoon kosher salt

¼ teaspoon coarsely ground black pepper

2 tablespoons balsamic vinegar,
   plus more if needed

1. Preheat the broiler. Rub both sides of the chops with a cut side of the garlic and sprinkle with the rosemary, salt, and pepper.

2. Place the chops on a rack in a broiling pan. Place the pan under the broiler in the position closest to the heat source; broil the chops 4 minutes. Brush the chops with 1 tablespoon of the balsamic; broil 1 minute. Turn the chops and broil 4 more minutes. Brush the chops with the remaining 1 tablespoon balsamic and broil 1 minute longer for medium-rare, or to the desired doneness.

3. Transfer the lamb to a warm platter. Skim and discard the fat from the drippings in the broiling pan. Serve the chops with the pan juices, or drizzle them with additional balsamic vinegar.

SERVES 4: About 240 calories, 26g protein, 14g carbohydrate, 8g fat (3g saturated), 0g fiber, 223mg sodium.

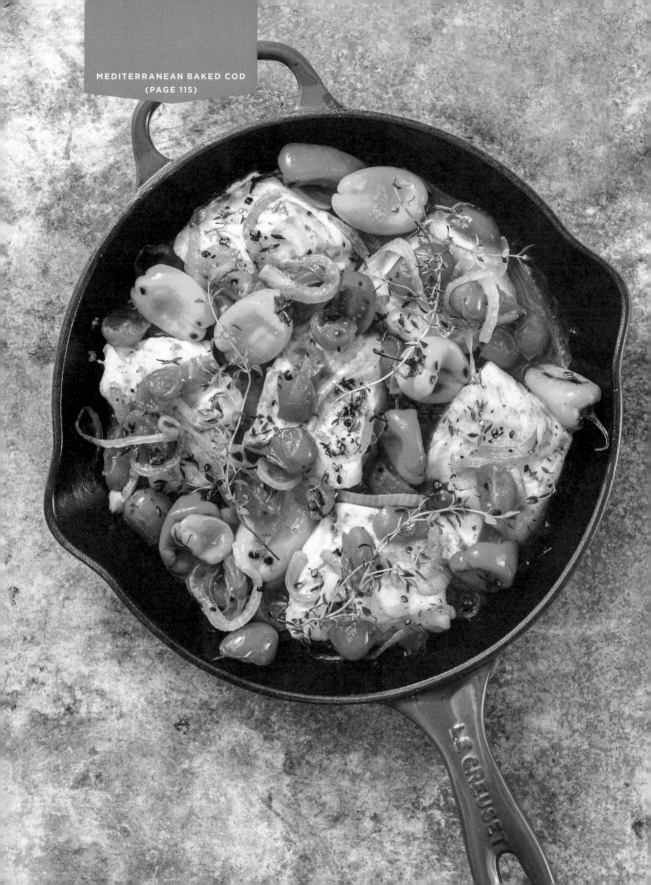

MEDITERRANEAN BAKED COD
(PAGE 115)

5 | Fish

What would a diet plan be without fish? Salmon, loaded with omega-3 fatty acids and antioxidants, is a pro dieter's choice. Here we roast it with green beans, tomatoes, and olives for a rich Mediterranean dish. Give it a New Orleans-style keto treatment with Creole flavors and crunchy almonds, and glaze it with a zippy soy-jalapeno mix.

Cod is a milder, leaner fish that roasts and steams beautifully. Baked in a parchment pouch with smoky bacon and cabbage, it's a dish you will crave! If you're not finding cod in your market, you could swap in tilapia, flounder, or another mild fish.

Roasted Shrimp and Poblano Salad gets a south-of-the-border touch with roasted chiles, avocado, radishes, and a tangy lime dressing. *Muy delicioso!*

Indian Tandoori Shrimp........................114

Mediterranean Baked Cod 115

Roasted Shrimp &
Poblano Salad 117

Roasted Salmon with
Tomatoes & Green Beans................118

Almond-Crusted Creole
Salmon 120

Cod, Cabbage & Bacon
in Parchment....................................121

Spicy Soy-Glazed Salmon 122

113

Indian Tandoori Shrimp

Be sure your grill is nice and hot to get the
characteristic char marks of a good tandoor.

~~~~~~

TOTAL: 20 MINUTES, PLUS MARINATING

~~~~~~

½ cup plain yogurt

1 large clove garlic, grated

2 teaspoons grated peeled fresh ginger

2 teaspoons garam masala

1 teaspoon ground turmeric

¼ teaspoon cayenne pepper

1 teaspoon finely grated lemon zest

Kosher salt and ground black pepper

**1 pound peeled and deveined large shrimp
(about 18)**

**3 tablespoons fresh lemon juice,
plus lemon wedges for serving**

**Very thinly sliced red onion and fresh
chopped cilantro, for serving**

1. In a large bowl, combine the yogurt, garlic, ginger, spices, lemon zest, and ¼ teaspoon each salt and pepper. Add the shrimp; toss to coat. Cover and refrigerate 30 minutes.

2. Preheat a grill or grill pan on medium-high. Toss the shrimp mixture with the lemon juice, then thread the shrimp onto skewers. Grill until just opaque throughout, 2 to 3 minutes per side.

3. Transfer the shrimp to a platter and top with sliced red onion and cilantro. Serve with lemon wedges.

SERVES 4: About 135 calories, 21g protein, 6g carbohydrates, 2.5g fat (1g saturated), 1g fiber, 955mg sodium.

Mediterranean Baked Cod

Steam-baking the cod keeps it moist and helps the herb
flavor infuse the fish. See photo on page 112.

PREP: 10 MINUTES   TOTAL: 25 MINUTES

1 tablespoon olive oil

1 medium onion, thinly sliced

6 ounces mini sweet peppers

Kosher salt

1 pint grape tomatoes, halved lengthwise

8 sprigs fresh thyme

1½ pounds cod fillets

¼ cup water

¼ teaspoon ground black pepper

1. Preheat the oven to 450°F.

2. In a 7- to 8-quart wide-bottomed oven-safe saucepot, heat the oil on medium-high. Cook the onion, sweet peppers, and ¼ teaspoon salt 5 minutes, or until the onions are almost tender, stirring occasionally.

3. Add the grape tomatoes and thyme; cook 2 minutes.

4. Add the cod fillets and water; sprinkle the cod with ¼ teaspoon salt and the pepper. Cover and bake for 15 minutes, or until the cod is cooked through. Discard the thyme sprigs and serve.

SERVES 4: About 205 calories, 32g protein, 8g carbohydrates, 5g fat (1g saturated), 1g fiber, 115mg sodium.

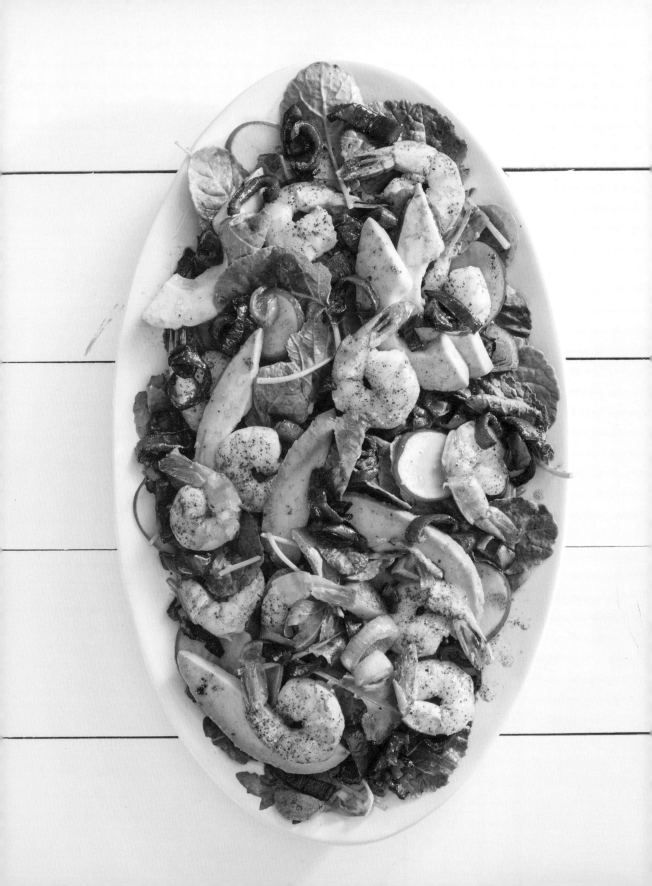

Roasted Shrimp & Poblano Salad

To check the ripeness of avocado, place it in the palm of your hand and gently tighten your hand. If the fruit gives a bit, it's ready, but if it feels soft, it's overripe.

PREP: 15 MINUTES   TOTAL: 40 MINUTES

2 medium shallots, sliced

3 poblano peppers, seeded and sliced crosswise

1 tablespoon canola oil

2 teaspoons chili powder

1 pound peeled and deveined large shrimp (about 18)

4 radishes, sliced

3 tablespoons fresh lime juice

½ teaspoon kosher salt

½ (5-ounce) container mixed greens

1 avocado, thinly sliced

1. Preheat the oven to 450°F. In a bowl, toss the shallots and poblanos with the oil and chili powder. Arrange them on a baking sheet; roast 20 minutes.

2. To same baking sheet, add the shrimp. Roast 5 minutes; cool slightly. Combine the shrimp mixture, radishes, lime juice, salt, and mixed greens. Top with avocado slices and serve.

SERVES 4: About 215 calories, 17g protein, 9g carbohydrates, 12g fat (2g saturated), 2g fiber, 940mg sodium.

TIP

To peel your own shrimp, use kitchen shears to cut down the back (the round side) of the shell and into the shrimp. Pull off the shell with your fingers and rinse away the dark vein.

Roasted Salmon with Tomatoes & Green Beans

Salmon is a keto superhero: Rich in healthy fats, a good source of protein—and it's satisfying and versatile.

PREP: 5 MINUTES   TOTAL: 25 MINUTES

6 ounces green beans, trimmed

¼ cup water

1 cup grape tomatoes

¼ cup pitted Kalamata olives

4 oil-packed anchovies, drained

1 tablespoon olive oil

Kosher salt and ground black pepper

2 skinless center-cut salmon fillets (6 ounces each)

1. Preheat the oven to 425°F. Heat a large oven-safe skillet on medium-high, add the green beans and water, cover, and cook, shaking the pan occasionally, 3 minutes. Drain the beans and transfer them to a bowl.

2. Wipe out the skillet. In a bowl, toss the beans with the grape tomatoes, olives, anchovies, and oil and lightly season with salt and pepper. Return to the skillet and roast 8 minutes.

3. Season the salmon fillets with salt and pepper and nestle them among the vegetables in the skillet. Roast until the salmon is just opaque throughout, 10 to 12 minutes.

SERVES 2: About 355 calories, 38g protein, 10g carbohydrates, 18g fat (3.5g saturated), 4g fiber, 1,105mg sodium.

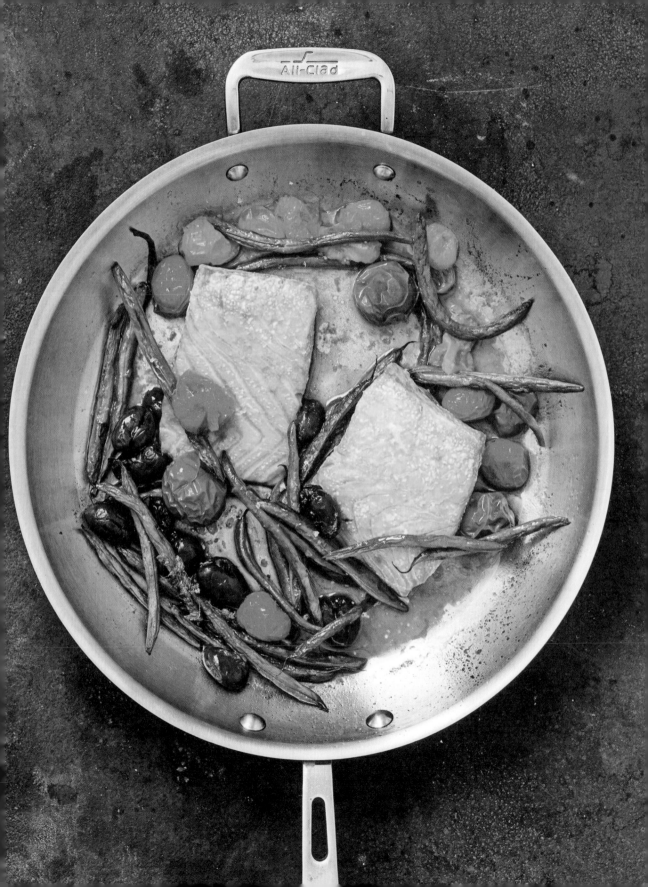

Almond-Crusted Creole Salmon

This yummy one pan dinner covers all the
weeknight bases for Keto: fast and easy, includes healthy fats
and protein, and you get extra crunch from almonds.

PREP: 10 MINUTES   TOTAL: 25 MINUTES

1 pound green beans, trimmed

1 tablespoon olive oil

½ teaspoon kosher salt

½ teaspoon ground black pepper

1 cup plain Greek yogurt

2 teaspoons Creole seasoning

1 teaspoon lemon zest

**4 skinless salmon fillets
   (6 ounces each)**

1 cup sliced almonds, coarsely chopped

Nonstick cooking spray

1. Preheat the oven to 450°F. Line a large
rimmed baking sheet with foil.

2. In a large bowl, toss the green beans with
the oil, salt, and pepper. Arrange on the baking
sheet and roast 10 minutes.

3. In a bowl, stir together the yogurt, Creole
seasoning, and lemon zest. Spread onto the
salmon fillets; top with sliced almonds. Push
the beans to one side of the baking sheet;
place salmon on other side. Spray the salmon
with nonstick cooking spray. Bake 12 minutes,
or until the salmon is cooked through and the
beans are tender.

SERVES 4: About 310 calories, 39g protein,
9g carbohydrates, 13g fat (2g saturated),
4g fiber, 540mg sodium.

TIP

Swap finely chopped pistachios or pecans
for the almonds.

Cod, Cabbage & Bacon In Parchment

Bacon and fish? You bet! Snowy white fish steams with wilted bacon-flecked cabbage for a delicious meal in a pouch.

PREP: 20 MINUTES TOTAL: 40 MINUTES

4 slices bacon, chopped

2 teaspoons vegetable oil

½ **head savoy cabbage (¾ pound),** thinly sliced (6 cups)

Kosher salt and ground black pepper

Pinch of dried thyme

4 thick pieces cod fillet (6 ounces each)

1 tablespoon butter, cut into very small pieces

1. Preheat the oven to 400°F and prepare four 12-inch squares of parchment or foil.

2. In a 12-inch skillet, cook the bacon on medium-low for 8 minutes or until browned. With a slotted spoon, transfer it to paper towels to drain. Discard the drippings from the skillet; wipe the skillet clean.

3. In the same skillet, heat the oil on high. Add the cabbage, ½ teaspoon salt, ¼ teaspoon pepper, and the thyme; cook, stirring, until the cabbage is tender. Stir in the bacon.

4. With tweezers, remove any bones from the cod. Place one-fourth of the cabbage mixture on one half of each parchment square. Place the fillets on top of the cabbage. Sprinkle the fillets with ⅛ teaspoon each of salt and pepper and evenly dot with the butter.

5. Fold the unfilled half of the parchment over the cod. To seal the packets, beginning at a corner where the parchment is folded, make ½-inch-wide folds, with each new fold overlapping the previous one, until the packet is completely sealed. The packets will resemble half circles. Place the packets on a jelly-roll pan. Bake 20 minutes (packets will puff up and brown). Cut the packets open to serve.

SERVES 4: About 250 calories, 35g protein, 5g carbohydrates, 10g fat (3g saturated), 3g fiber, 576mg sodium.

Spicy Soy-Glazed Salmon

This spicy roasted celery and green onion relish adds
savory satisfying crunch to simple salmon.

PREP: 15 MINUTES   **TOTAL: 30 MINUTES**

5 stalks celery, very thinly sliced

1 bunch green onions, thinly sliced

4 jalapeño chilies, seeded and thinly sliced

1 tablespoon vegetable oil

⅛ teaspoon kosher salt

4 skinless salmon fillets (6 ounces each)

2 tablespoons lower-sodium soy sauce

Steamed bok choy, for serving

**¼ cup unsalted peanuts, chopped,
and sliced green onions, for garnish**

1. Preheat the oven to 450°F. On a large rimmed baking sheet, toss the celery, green onions, jalapeños, oil, and salt. Roast 15 minutes, stirring twice.

2. Place the salmon in a 2-quart square baking dish and drizzle with the soy sauce. Roast the salmon alongside the vegetables 12 minutes, or until just opaque. Serve the salmon with the celery mixture and steamed bok choy. Garnish the salmon with peanuts and green onions.

SERVES 4: About 335 calories, 39g protein, 11g carbohydrates, 14g fat (3g saturated), 4g fiber, 690mg sodium.

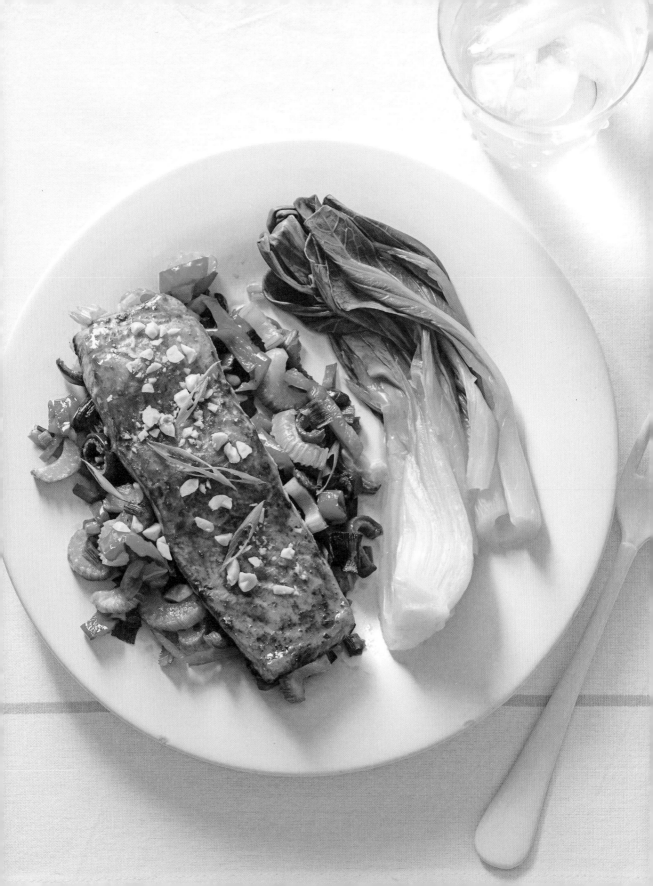

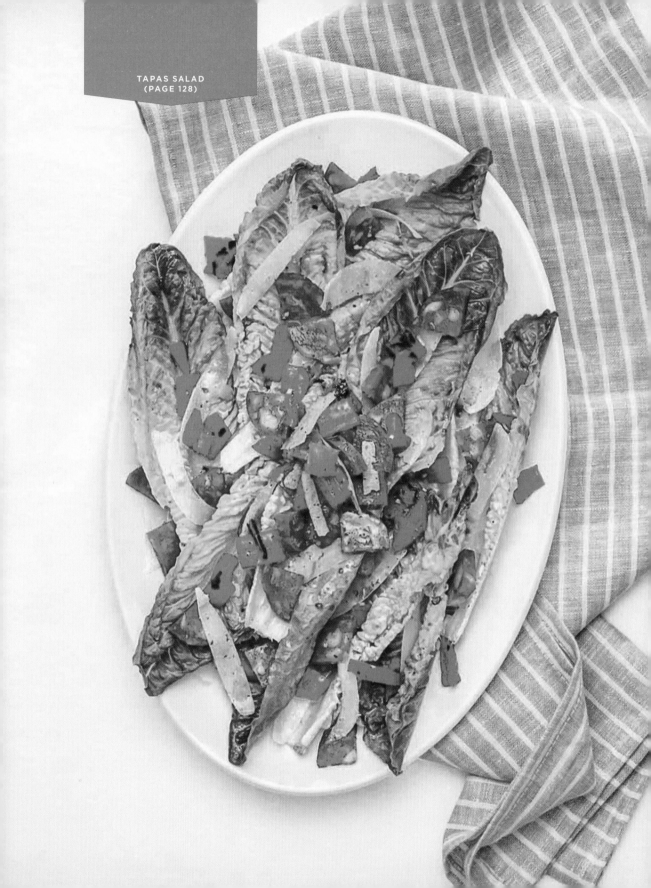

TAPAS SALAD
(PAGE 128)

6 | Vegetables & Salads

Who said you can't have veggies on the keto diet? Here we offer plenty of low-carb options. Feta-Dill Greek Caesar features romaine hearts that are quickly charred and topped with a creamy lemony dressing and crunchy sunflower seeds. You can make a meal of chorizo and manchego-laden Tapas Salad. In an updated riff on spinach salad, Wilted Kale Salad features bacon, onions, and goat cheese. Don't miss the Lemony Brussels Sprouts Salad studded with smoked almonds and shredded pecorino cheese.

Veggie sides like Sautéed Spinach, Nutty Green Beans & Asparagus with Bacon, and Asparagus with Eggs Mimosa, keep it simple and delicious. For more veggie options see the Roasting Vegetables chart on page 95.

Feta-Dill Greek Caesar 126

Tapas Salad 128

Wilted Kale Salad 128

Sautéed Spinach with Garlic 129

Lemony Brussels Sprout Salad 131

Nutty Green Beans &
Asparagus with Bacon 132

Asparagus with Eggs Mimosa 135

Buffalo Chicken Cobb Salad 136

Warm Goat Cheese Salad 138

Ranch Dressing 139

Pesto 139

Feta-Dill Greek Caesar

Feta does double duty here replacing the creaminess of the egg and the salt of the anchovies. If you love anchovies, omit the salt and add a few.

PREP: 10 MINUTES   TOTAL: 15 MINUTES

4 ounces feta cheese

⅔ cup extra-virgin olive oil

⅓ cup plain Greek yogurt

3 tablespoons fresh lemon juice

1 clove garlic

¼ teaspoon kosher salt

¼ teaspoon ground black pepper

¼ cup packed fresh dill, chopped

3 romaine lettuce hearts

¼ cup roasted sunflower seeds, for serving

1. Preheat a grill or grill pan on medium heat.

2. In a blender or food processor, puree the feta, oil, Greek yogurt, lemon juice, garlic, salt, and pepper. Transfer to medium bowl; stir in the dill.

3. Cut the romaine lettuce hearts in half lengthwise; grill until charred in spots, about 2 minutes per side. Serve immediately, drizzled with the yogurt dressing and sprinkled with roasted sunflower seeds.

SERVES 6: About 325 calories, 6g protein, 5g carbohydrates, 32g fat (7g saturated), 1g fiber, 265 mg sodium.

TIP

Trim an inch off the base of your romaine hearts to release the leaves all at once.

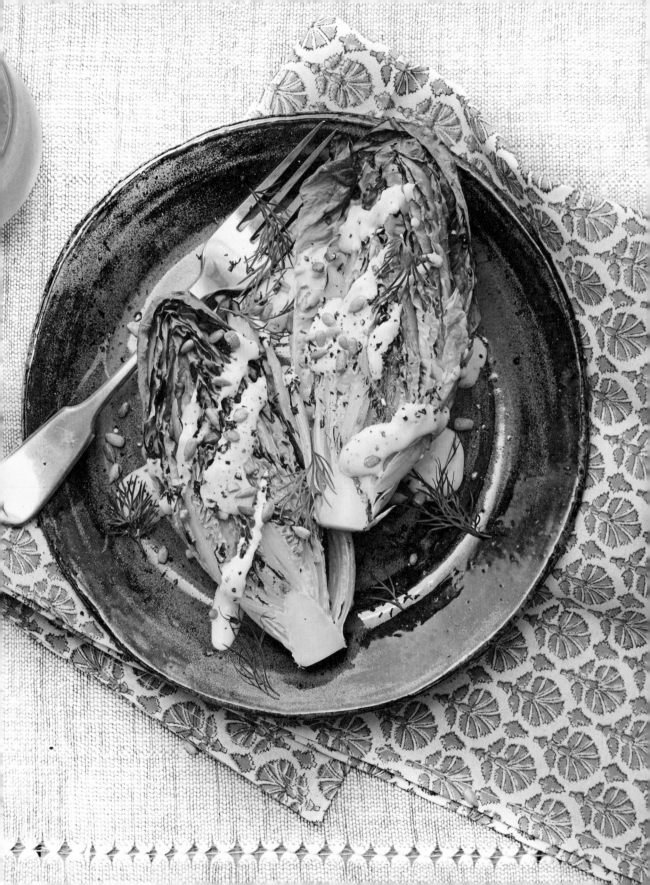

Tapas Salad

Manchego cheese and cured chorizo star in this keto-friendly Spanish sampler. See photo on page 124.

~~~~~~
TOTAL: 15 MINUTES
~~~~~~

3 tablespoons extra-virgin olive oil

2 tablespoons sherry vinegar

1 clove garlic, crushed with a press

Kosher salt and ground black pepper

1 cup packed shaved Manchego cheese

4 ounces Spanish chorizo, cut into quarters lengthwise, then thinly sliced

½ cup roasted red peppers, chopped

2 romaine lettuce hearts, leaves separated

1. In large bowl, whisk together the oil, sherry vinegar, garlic, and salt and pepper to taste. Add the Manchego, chorizo, and roasted red peppers. Toss well.

2. Arrange the romaine leaves on a serving platter. Top with cheese-chorizo mixture.

SERVES 4: About 305 calories, 11g protein, 5g carbohydrates, 26g fat (9g saturated), 2g fiber, 640mg sodium.

Wilted Kale Salad

Hearty good-for-you greens get a boost of rich flavor from sautéed bacon and onion and a sprinkling of tangy goat cheese.

~~~~~~
TOTAL: 20 MINUTES
~~~~~~

6 slices bacon, chopped

1 cup chopped onion

7 cups thinly sliced kale leaves

2 tablespoons red wine vinegar

¼ teaspoon kosher salt

¼ teaspoon ground black pepper

½ cup crumbled goat cheese

1. In a 12-inch skillet on medium, cook the bacon 8 minutes or until browned. Stir in the onion; cook 8 minutes, or until the onion is tender.

2. In a large bowl, toss the sliced kale leaves with the vinegar, salt, and pepper, and then with the bacon mixture.

3. Top with crumbled goat cheese and serve.

SERVES 4: About 245 calories, 9g protein, 7g carbohydrates, 20g fat (8g saturated), 2g fiber, 478mg sodium.

Sautéed Spinach with Garlic

Here's a back-pocket recipe you'll use again and again. You can swap in any leafy green (remove tough stems from the heartier ones like kale and mustard greens) and just cook until tender. If you like a bit of heat add ¼ teaspoon crushed red pepper along with the garlic.

PREP: 5 MINUTES TOTAL: 10 MINUTES

1 tablespoon olive oil

2 cloves garlic, crushed with the side of a chef's knife

2 bags (10 ounces each) fresh spinach, well rinsed

1 tablespoon fresh lemon juice

¼ teaspoon kosher salt

1. In a 5- to 6-quart saucepot, heat the oil on medium-high until hot. Add the garlic and cook 1 minute, or until golden, stirring continuously.

2. Add the spinach, with water clinging to the leaves, to the pot in 2 or 3 batches; cook 2 minutes, or until all the spinach fits in the saucepot. Cover and cook 2 to 3 minutes longer, or just until the spinach wilts, stirring once. Remove from the heat. Stir in the lemon juice and salt.

SERVES 4: About 45 calories, 4g protein, 1g carbohydrates, 4g fat (1g saturated), 12g fiber, 305mg sodium.

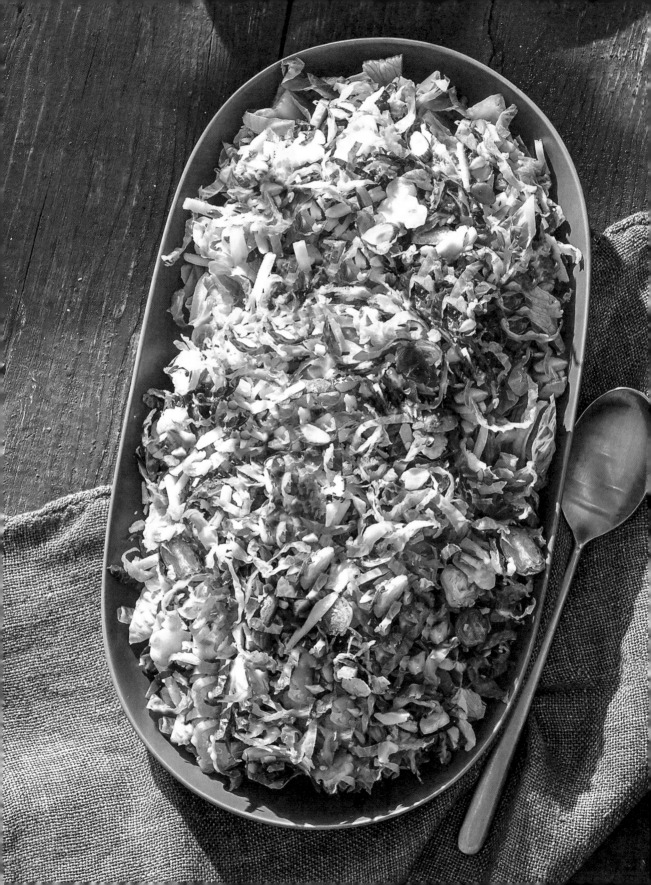

Lemony Brussels Sprout Salad

Brussels sprouts are tiny but mighty nutritional powerhouses. Like their cruciferous cousins (broccoli, cabbage, and cauliflower) they deliver more than the 100 percent of the recommended daily allowance for Vitamins C and K, a healthy dose of fiber, and antioxidants.

PREP: 20 MINUTES   TOTAL: 25 MINUTES

¼ cup fresh lemon juice

3 tablespoons extra-virgin olive oil

½ teaspoon kosher salt

¼ teaspoon ground black pepper

1 pound Brussels sprouts, trimmed and very thinly sliced

1 small head romaine lettuce, chopped

⅓ cup packed grated ricotta salata or Pecorino Romano cheese

½ cup smoked almonds, chopped

1. In a large bowl, whisk together the lemon juice, oil, salt, and pepper; add the Brussels sprouts and toss until well coated. Let stand at least 10 minutes or up to 2 hours.

2. When ready to serve, add the romaine, ricotta salata, and almonds to the bowl with the Brussels sprouts; toss to combine.

SERVES 8: About 145 calories, 5g protein, 8g carbohydrates, 12g fat (2g saturated), 3g fiber, 292mg sodium.

TIP

The easiest way to thinly shave Brussels sprouts is on a mandolin. Leave the stem on and, holding the stem, carefully slice from top toward the stem. You can also use the food processor; simply pile trimmed sprouts into the feed tube.

Nutty Green Beans & Asparagus with Bacon

Want to make asparagus even more delicious and keto-friendly?
Add crisp bacon and pecans and toss with a shallot-lemon dressing.

PREP: 20 MINUTES TOTAL: 30 MINUTES

1 large lemon

Kosher salt

8 ounces green beans, trimmed

1 pound asparagus, trimmed

3 slices bacon, chopped

1 medium shallot, finely chopped

½ teaspoon kosher salt

½ teaspoon ground black pepper

¼ cup chopped pecans

1. From the lemon, grate all the zest and squeeze ¼ cup juice; set aside.

2. Heat a large covered saucepot of salted water to boiling on high. Add the green beans; cook 1 minute. Add the asparagus; cook 2 to 4 minutes, or until the vegetables are tender. Drain well. Return the vegetables to the pot and set aside.

3. While the water is heating, in a 10-inch skillet, cook the bacon on medium 8 minutes, or until crisp, stirring occasionally. With a slotted spoon, transfer the cooked bacon to a small plate. To the rendered fat in the skillet, add the shallots; cook 3 minutes, stirring occasionally. Whisk in the reserved lemon juice, salt, and pepper.

4. In the pot used to cook the vegetables, toss the shallot mixture with the vegetables; transfer them to a serving platter. Top with bacon, pecans, and the reserved lemon zest.

SERVES 4: About 155 calories, 5g protein, 8g carbohydrates, 12g fat (3 g saturated), 3g fiber, 250mg sodium.

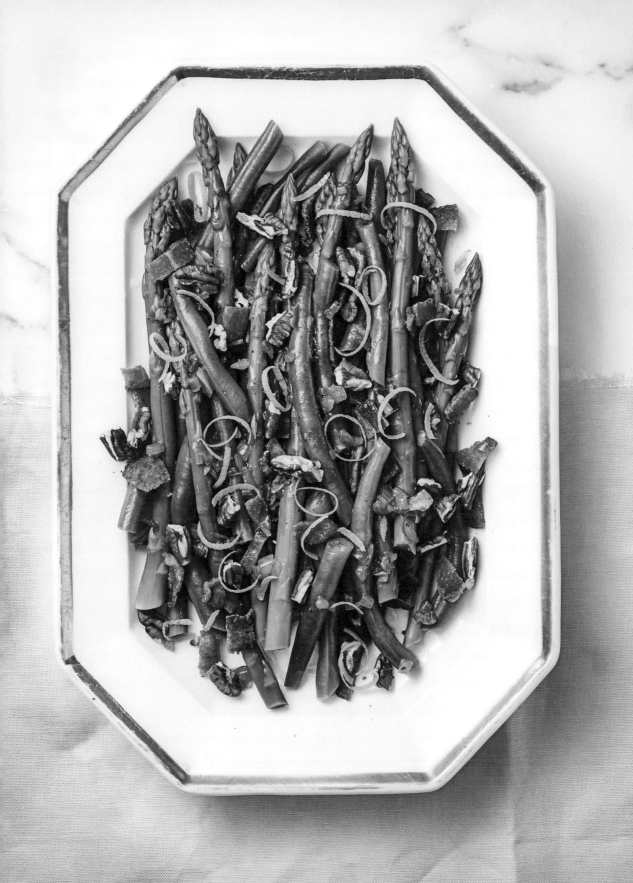

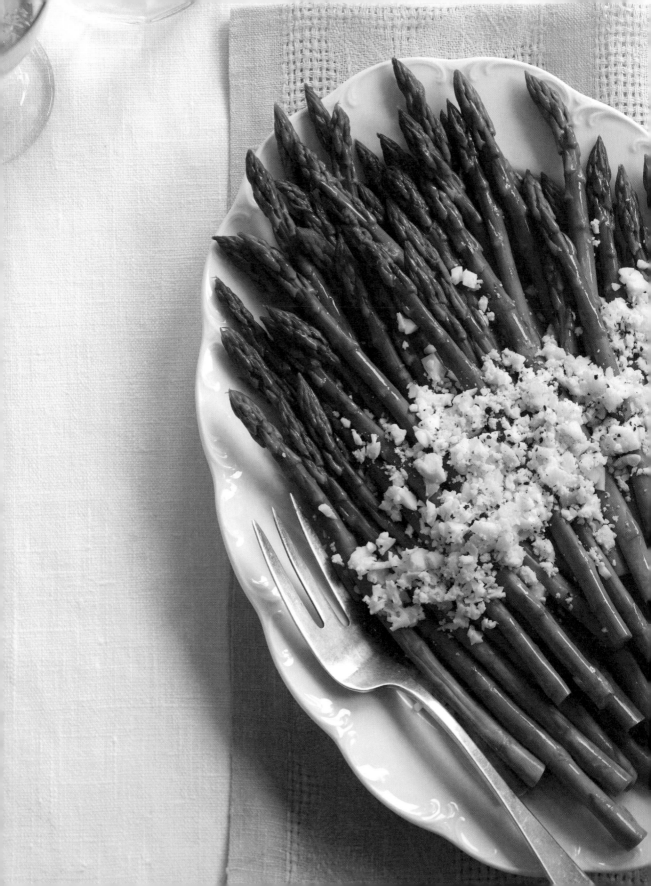

Asparagus with Eggs Mimosa

Bright green asparagus gets a shower of grated egg and lemon zest for springtime on a plate. You can prepare the asparagus, dressing, and eggs ahead of time—just dress at the last minute to keep the colors vibrant.

PREP: 20 MINUTES   TOTAL: 35 MINUTES

3 large eggs

2 pounds asparagus, trimmed

¼ cup water

1 lemon

3 tablespoons extra-virgin olive oil

2 tablespoons red wine vinegar

1 tablespoon snipped fresh chives

½ teaspoon kosher salt

½ teaspoon ground black pepper

1. In a 2-quart saucepan, combine the eggs and enough cold water to cover. Heat to boiling on high. Remove from heat. Cover and let stand 14 minutes. Rinse the eggs with cold water until cool, then peel. Eggs may be hard-cooked and refrigerated up to 3 days ahead.

2. Meanwhile, cook the asparagus: Arrange the asparagus in even layer in a microwave-safe 8 × 8-inch baking dish. Add the water. Cover with vented plastic wrap and microwave on High 5 minutes. The asparagus may be cooked, cooled, and refrigerated in an airtight container up to 2 days.

3. From the lemon, grate ¼ teaspoon zest; set aside. Squeeze 1 tablespoon juice into a small bowl. Add the oil, vinegar, chives, salt, and pepper to the bowl with the lemon juice; whisk to combine.

4. To serve, arrange the asparagus on a serving platter. Drizzle with vinaigrette. Coarsely grate the hard-cooked eggs over the asparagus and garnish with reserved lemon zest.

SERVES 6: About 135 calories, 6g protein, 3g carbohydrates, 11g total fat (2g saturated), 2g fiber, 255mg sodium.

Buffalo Chicken Cobb Salad

The classic wing flavors pair up with lettuce, tomatoes, and eggs and get dressed with a silky Avocado-Buttermilk Ranch Dressing. Looking to up your ratios? Add an ounce of crumbled blue cheese to each serving.

PREP: 35 MINUTES   TOTAL: 40 MINUTES

1 cup buttermilk

1 ripe small avocado

2 tablespoons fresh lemon juice

1 clove garlic

¾ teaspoon kosher salt

¾ teaspoon ground black pepper

2 tablespoons chopped fresh dill

1 tablespoon snipped fresh chives

2 cups rotisserie chicken meat cut into bite-size pieces

⅓ cup cayenne pepper hot sauce

1 teaspoon distilled white vinegar

6 hard-cooked eggs

3 stalks celery

3 small tomatoes

1 head butter lettuce or Boston lettuce

1. In a blender, puree buttermilk, avocado, lemon juice, garlic, kosher salt, and ground black pepper until smooth. Transfer to a container; stir in chopped fresh dill and snipped fresh chives. Makes 1 cup.

2. In a medium bowl, toss the chicken with the hot sauce and vinegar until well coated.

3. Slice the eggs crosswise and thinly slice the celery; cut the tomatoes into wedges or slices. Separate the lettuce leaves; arrange them on a large serving platter. Top with the eggs, celery, tomatoes, and chicken. Drizzle with the dressing. Refrigerate the remaining dressing for another use.

SERVES 6: About 200 calories, 16g protein, 8g carbohydrates, 14g fat (4g saturated), 2g fiber, 880mg sodium.

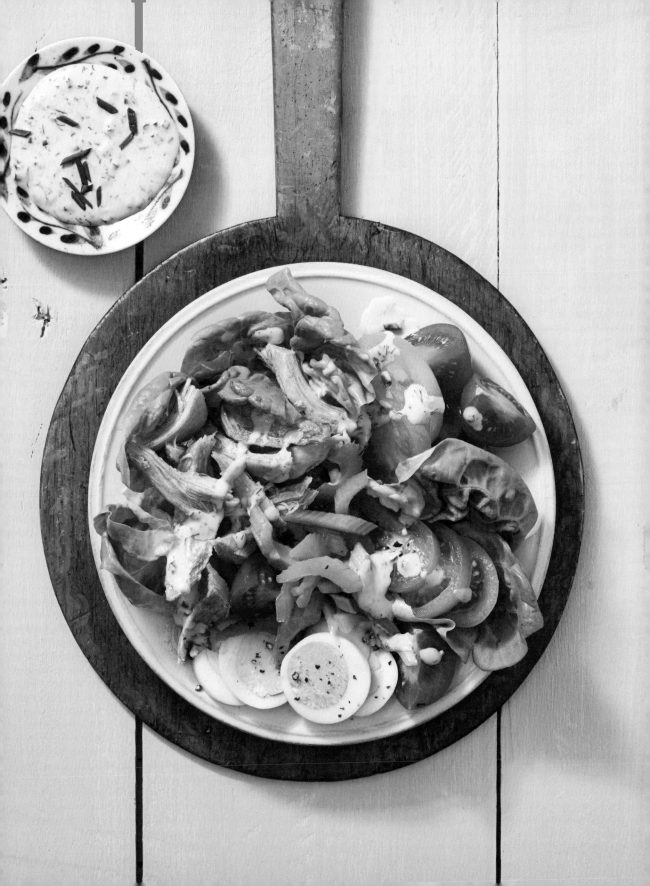

Warm Goat Cheese Salad

Yes diet salads can be delicious! Goat cheese gets rolled in ground almonds and baked for extra crunch. It's perfect to start a meal—or have a double serving for lunch!

PREP: 15 MINUTES   TOTAL: 25 MINUTES

¼ cup ground almonds

1 tablespoon chopped fresh parsley

1 tablespoon olive oil

Coarsely ground black pepper

1 log (5 to 6 ounces) mild goat cheese

¼ cup wine vinegar

1 tablespoon Dijon mustard

¾ teaspoon kosher salt

8 ounces mixed baby salad greens

1. Preheat the oven to 425°F. In a small bowl, stir the almonds, parsley, oil, and pepper until well blended. Slice the goat cheese crosswise into 6 equal disks. Place them on waxed paper; coat the disks in the almond mixture, patting the nuts to cover them evenly.

2. Place the coated cheese disks on a baking sheet and bake until the nuts are golden, 8 to 10 minutes.

3. Meanwhile, in a jar with a tight-fitting lid, combine wine vinegar, Dijon mustard, kosher salt, and ½ teaspoon coarsely ground black pepper. Secure the lid and shake the dressing until well blended. Makes ¾ cup dressing and can be refrigerated up to 1 week.

4. In a large bowl, toss the salad greens with 3 tablespoons of the vinaigrette to coat. Divide the greens among 6 salad plates and top each with a warm goat cheese disk.

SERVES 6: About 180 calories, 7g protein, 5g carbohydrates, 15g fat (6g saturated), 1g fiber, 265mg sodium.

Ranch Dressing

Arguably America's favorite for dipping and dressing, this keto version gets enriched with mayo and Greek yogurt. Stir in some snipped chives if you like.

TOTAL: 10 MINUTES

¾ cup full-fat buttermilk

½ cup mayonnaise

⅓ cup Greek yogurt

2 tablespoons fresh lemon juice

1 tablespoon Dijon mustard

1 clove garlic

¾ teaspoon kosher salt

¼ teaspoon ground black pepper

½ cup loosely packed fresh parsley

2 tablespoons snipped fresh chives

1. In a blender, puree the buttermilk, mayonnaise, Greek yogurt, lemon juice, mustard, garlic, salt, and pepper until smooth.

2. Add the parsley and chives; pulse until just finely chopped. Keeps, refrigerated, for up to 2 weeks. Dressing may separate; stir before using. Makes about 2¼ cups.

EACH TABLESPOON: About 25 calories, 0g protein, 1g carbohydrate, 3g fat (0g saturated), 0g fiber, 77mg sodium.

Pesto

Pesto is your meal maker. Toss it with zoodles, use it as a marinade or topping for any cooked meat or fish, or stir into Greek yogurt for a dip. When basil is in season, make a double batch and freeze some.

TOTAL: 15 MINUTES

3 cups loosely packed fresh basil leaves

1 large garlic clove, crushed with a press

½ cup extra-virgin olive oil

¼ cup grated Parmesan cheese

¼ cup toasted pine nuts

2 teaspoons fresh lemon juice

¼ teaspoon ground black pepper

In a food processor or blender, pulse the basil, garlic, oil, Parmesan, pine nuts, lemon juice, and pepper until smooth. Keeps refrigerated 3 days. Makes ¾ cup.

EACH TABLESPOON: About 110 calories, 1g protein, 1g carbohydrate, 11g fat (2g saturated), 0g fiber, 31mg sodium.

Index
Note: Page numbers in *italics* indicate photos separate from recipes.

A

Almonds. *See* Nuts and seeds
Appetizers and snacks, 33–51
  about: overview of recipes, 33
  Artichoke Dip, 40
  Asian Garden Veggie Rolls, 37
  Bacon Cheddar Bombs, 48
  Caesar Deviled Eggs, 45
  Cauliflower "Popcorn" (and fun flavors), *38–39*
  Cheddar Crisps, 36
  Chili Lime Cauliflower "Popcorn," 39
  Chocolate Pudding Bombs, 50
  Classic Deviled Eggs, 45
  Coconut Lime Cheesecake Bombs, 51
  Crunchy Curry Deviled Eggs, 45
  Deviled Eggs (and fun flavors), *10*, 44–45
  Everything Cheese Balls (and fun flavors), *42–43*
  Frico Cups, *32*, 36
  Grape Tomato, Olive & Feta Salad, *32*, 35
  Guacamole Deviled Eggs, 44
  Ham & Cheese Deviled Eggs, 44
  Hot 'N' Smoky Ricotta (and fun flavors), 41
  Marinated Mixed Olives, 40
  Miso-Ginger Deviled Eggs, 45
  Parmesan Crisps, 36
  Peanut Butter Bombs, 49
  Pesto-Bacon Deviled Eggs, 44
  Pimiento-Cheese Deviled Eggs, *10*, 44
  Red Pepper-Basil Veggie Rolls, 37
  Savory Dill Cheese Balls, 43
  Savory Herb Ricotta, 41
  Sesame Smoked Salmon Bombs, 46
  Smoky Chipotle Deviled Eggs, 45
  Smoky Manchego Bombs, 47
  Spiced Citrus Ricotta, 41
  Sweet & Spicy Cheese Balls, 43
  Tomato & Mozzarella Bites, *34–35*
  Truffle Cauliflower "Popcorn," 39
  Veggie Chili Veggie Rolls, 37
  Veggie Rolls (with variations), 37
  Zippy Pear Veggie Rolls, 37
Artichokes
  Artichoke Dip, 40
  Chicken with Creamy Spinach & Artichokes, 62
Asian Garden Veggie Rolls, 37
Asparagus
  about: roasting, 95
  Asparagus & Romano Frittata, 27
  Asparagus with Eggs Mimosa, *134–135*
  Bacon & Eggs Over Asparagus, 103
  Nutty Green Beans & Asparagus with Bacon, *132–133*
Avocados
  about: testing ripeness and ripening, 26
  Huevos Rancheros, 26
  Salsa-Avocado Omelet Filling, 24

B

Bacon. *See* Pork
Basil
  Chicken Caprese, 75
  Pesto, 139
  Red Pepper-Basil Veggie Rolls, 37
  Tomato & Mozzarella Bites, *34–35*
Beef
  Chimichurri Strip Steak, 83
  Coffee-Rubbed Beef Tenderloin, 85
  Feta & Mint Mini Meatloaves, *96–97*
  Grilled Plumb Tomatoes with, 83
  Grilled Southwest Steak Salad, 82
  Korean Beef Lettuce Wraps, *92–93*
  Lebanese Kafta Kebabs, 110
  Seared Steak with Blistered Tomatoes, 94
  Soy-Braised Beef & Tomato-Mint Salad, *86–87*
  Sweet Pepper Sauce for, 85
  Thai Steak & Pear Salad, *90–91*
  Two-Step Slow-Cooked Brisket, *88–89*
  Wild-Mushroom Beef Brisket, *80*, 84
Berry Blast Smoothie, 30
Blender, 13
Blood ketone meter/test, 11
Bombs. *See* Appetizers and snacks
Breakfast, 15–31
  about: fillings for omelets, 24–25; overview of recipes, 15
  Asparagus & Romano Frittata, 27
  Basic Omelets (and fillings), 24–25
  Berry Blast Smoothie, 30
  Chive & Goat Cheese Frittata, 27
  Crustless Quiche Lorraine, *28–29*
  Green Light Juice, 31
  Huevos Rancheros, 26
  Lemon Cheesecake Smoothie, 31
  Lox Scrambled Eggs, *16–17*
  Scrambled Eggs with Cream Cheese, 18
  Spinach & Prosciutto Frittata Muffins, *22–23*
  Summer Squash Frittata, *20–21*
  Tuscan Sausage & Kale Frittata, *14*, 19
Broccoli
  about: roasting, 95
  Grilled Pork with Charred Harissa Broccoli, *98*
Broths, 12
Brussels sprouts
  about: roasting, 95; shaving, 131
  Lemony Brussels Sprout Salad, *130–131*
Buffalo Chicken Cobb Salad, *136–137*

C

Cabbage, cod and bacon in parchment, 121
Caesar Deviled Eggs, 45
Carbohydrates
  energy from fat vs., 8
  hidden sources of, 12
  ketosis and, 8, 11
  ratios for keto diet, 9
  removing cues from kitchen, 12
  tracking, net vs. total carbs, 11
Cauliflower
  about: roasting, 95; tips for using stems, 39
  Cauliflower "Popcorn" (and fun flavors), *38–39*
Challenges of keto diet, 8–9
Cheese
  Bacon Cheddar Bombs, 48
  Cheddar Crisps, 36
  Chicken Caprese, 75
  Chocolate Pudding Bombs, 50
  Coconut Lime Cheesecake Bombs, 51
  eggs with. *See* Eggs
  Everything Cheese Balls (and fun flavors), *42–43*
  Feta & Mint Mini Meatloaves, *96–97*
  Frico Cups, *32*, 36
  Ham & Cheese Deviled Eggs, 44
  Hot 'N' Smoky Ricotta (and fun flavors), 41
  Lemon Cheesecake Smoothie, 31
  Parmesan Crisps, 36
  Peanut Butter Bombs, 49
  Pimiento-Cheese Deviled Eggs, *10*, 44
  salads with. *See* Salads
  Savory Dill Cheese Balls, 43
  Savory Herb Ricotta, 41
  Sesame Smoked Salmon Bombs, 46
  Smoky Manchego Bombs, 47
  Spiced Citrus Ricotta, 41
  Sweet & Spicy Cheese Balls, 43
  Tomato & Mozzarella Bites, *34–35*
  Veggie Rolls (with variations), 37
Chicken. *See* Poultry
Chili Lime Cauliflower "Popcorn," 39
Chimichurri Strip Steak, 83
Chipotle Orange Chicken, *72–73*
Chive & Goat Cheese Frittata, 27
Chocolate
  Chocolate Pudding Bombs, 50
  Peanut Butter Bombs, 49
Chorizo. *See* Sausage
Cilantro-Lime Chicken, 74
Citrus
  Chili Lime Cauliflower "Popcorn," 39
  Chipotle Orange Chicken, *72–73*
  Cilantro-Lime Chicken, 74
  Coconut Lime Cheesecake Bombs, 51
  Lemon Cheesecake Smoothie, 31
  Lemony Brussels Sprout Salad, *130–131*
  Lemony Herb Roast Chicken, *64–65*
  Moroccan Chicken with Preserved Lemons & Olives, *78–79*
  Spiced Citrus Ricotta, 41
Coconut Lime Cheesecake Bombs, 51
Cod. *See* Fish
Coffee-Rubbed Beef Tenderloin, 85
Creamy Mushroom Omelet Filling, 24
Crispy Chicken with White Wine Pan Sauce, *52*, 57
Crunchy Curry Deviled Eggs, 45
Crustless Quiche Lorraine, *28–29*

D

Dairy, friendly to diet, 13
Dill cheese balls, 43
Drinks
  about: electrolyte importance, 8, 9; keto diet and, 9–11, 12
  Berry Blast Smoothie, 30
  Green Light Juice, 31
  Lemon Cheesecake Smoothie, 31

E

Eggplant, roasting, 95
Eggs
  about: boiling, 45; fillings for omelets, 24–25; golden yolks without green tint around, 45

Asparagus & Romano Frittata, 27

Asparagus with Eggs Mimosa, *134–135*

Bacon & Eggs Over Asparagus, 103

Basic Omelets (and fillings), 24–25

Buffalo Chicken Cobb Salad, 136–*137*

Caesar Deviled Eggs, 45

Chive & Goat Cheese Frittata, 27

Classic Deviled Eggs, 45

Creamy Mushroom Omelet Filling, 24

Crunchy Curry Deviled Eggs, 45

Crustless Quiche Lorraine, *28–29*

Deviled Eggs (and fun flavors), *10*, 44–45

Garden-Vegetable Omelet Filling, 25

Guacamole Deviled Eggs, 44

Ham & Cheese Deviled Eggs, 44

Huevos Rancheros, 26

Lox Scrambled Eggs, *16–17*

Miso-Ginger Deviled Eggs, 45

Pesto-Bacon Deviled Eggs, 44

Pimiento-Cheese Deviled Eggs, *10*, 44

Red Pepper & Goat Cheese Omelet Filling, 25

Salsa-Avocado Omelet Filling, 24

Scrambled Eggs with Cream Cheese, 18

Smoky Chipotle Deviled Eggs, 45

Spinach & Prosciutto Frittata Muffins, *22–23*

Summer Squash Frittata, *20–21*

Tuscan Sausage & Kale Frittata, *14*, 19

Western Omelet Filling, 25

Electrolytes, 8, 9

Equipment to ease tasks, 13

Espresso, in Chocolate Pudding Bombs, 50

Exercise, 11

F

Fat
  energy from burning, 8
  ketosis and, 8. *See also* Ketosis
  ratios for keto diet, 9

Fats and oils, to avoid and to use, 12

Fennel, roasting, 95

Fiery Kung Pao Chicken, 68–69

Fish, 113–123
  about: friendly to diet, 12; overview of recipes, 113; peeling shrimp, 117
  Almond-Crusted Creole Salmon, 120

Cod, Cabbage & Bacon in Parchment, 121

Indian Tandoori Shrimp, 114

Lox Scrambled Eggs, *16–17*

Mediterranean Baked Cod, *112*, 115

Roasted Salmon with Tomatoes & Green Beans, 118–*119*

Roasted Shrimp & Poblano Salad, *116–117*

Sesame Smoked Salmon Bombs, 46

Spicy Soy-Glazed Salmon, *122–123*

Fluids, drinking, 9–11

Food processor, 13

Food scale, 13

Foods, to include and avoid in diet, 12

Frico Cups, *32*, 36

Fruits, low-carb, friendly to diet, 13

G

Garden-Vegetable Omelet Filling, 25

Ginger, in Miso-Ginger Deviled Eggs, 45

Glazed Bacon-Wrapped Turkey Breast, *70–71*

Glazed Rosemary Lamb Chops, 111

Grape Tomato, Olive & Feta Salad, *32*, 35

Green beans
  about: roasting, 95
  Almond-Crusted Creole Salmon, 120
  Grilled Pork Tenderloin with Grainy Mustard Vinaigrette, 104–105
  Nutty Green Beans & Asparagus with Bacon, 132–*133*
  Pancetta Chicken, 66
  Roasted Salmon with Tomatoes & Green Beans, 118–*119*

Green Light Juice, 31

Grilled Plumb Tomatoes, 83

Grilled Pork Tenderloin & Peppers, *100–101*

Grilled Pork Tenderloin with Grainy Mustard Vinaigrette, 104–105

Grilled Pork with Charred Harissa Broccoli, *98*

Grilled Southwest Steak Salad, 82

Guacamole Deviled Eggs, 44

H

Ham & Cheese Deviled Eggs, 44

Herbs and spices, 12

Hot 'N' Smoky Ricotta (and fun flavors), 41

Huevos Rancheros, 26

I

Indian Tandoori Shrimp, 114

K

Kale
  Tuscan Sausage & Kale Frittata, *14*, 19
  Wilted Kale Salad, 128

Kebabs. *See* Skewers

Keto diet
  challenges of, 8–9
  defined, 8
  exercise, physical activity and, 11
  fluid intake during, 9–11
  foods to remove from kitchen/ diet, 12
  ketosis and, 8, 11
  other health ideas, 11
  ratios of macronutrients (macros), 9
  starting, 9
  for weight loss, 7, 8, 9, 11, 13
  whole foods friendly to, 12–13

"Keto flu," 8–9

Ketosis
  defined, 8
  how it happens, 8
  knowing if body is in, 11
  other ideas to maintain, 11
  testing to see if in, 11

Kitchen, preparing
  equipment to ease tasks, 13
  meal planning, 13
  removing carb cues, 12
  whole foods to stock, 12–13

Knives, 13

Korean Beef Lettuce Wraps, *92–93*

Kung Pao chicken, fiery, 68–69

L

Lamb
  Glazed Rosemary Lamb Chops, 111
  Lebanese Kafta Kebabs, 110

Lebanese Kafta Kebabs, 110

Lemon and lime. *See* Citrus

Lettuce wraps, Korean beef, *92–93*

Lighter Chicken Cacciatore, *60–61*

Lox Scrambled Eggs, *16–17*

M

Macronutrients (macros), ratios of, 9

Marinated Mixed Olives, 40

Meal planning, 13

Meatloaves, feta and mint, *96–97*

Meat/poultry, friendly to diet, 12. *See also* Poultry

Meat recipes, overview, 81. *See also specific meats*

Mediterranean Baked Cod, *112*, 115

Mint
  Feta & Mint Mini Meatloaves, *96–97*
  Soy-Braised Beef & Tomato-Mint Salad, *86–87*

Miso-Ginger Deviled Eggs, 45

Moroccan Chicken with Preserved Lemons & Olives, *78–79*

Mushrooms
  Creamy Mushroom Omelet Filling, 24
  Mushroom Chicken Skillet with Herbed Cream Sauce, *58–59*
  Rosemary-Truffle Sauce, 107
  Truffle Cauliflower "Popcorn," 39
  Western Omelet Filling, 25
  Wild-Mushroom Beef Brisket, 80, 84

Mustard vinaigrette, 105

N

Nigerian Peanutty Suya Skewers, 56

Nuts and seeds
  about: friendly to diet, 12
  Almond-Crusted Creole Salmon, 120
  Nigerian Peanutty Suya Skewers, 56
  Nutty Green Beans & Asparagus with Bacon, 132–*133*
  Peanut Butter Bombs, 49
  Sesame Smoked Salmon Bombs, 46

O

Olives
  Grape Tomato, Olive & Feta Salad, *32*, 35
  Marinated Mixed Olives, 40
  Moroccan Chicken with Preserved Lemons & Olives, *78–79*

Onions, roasting, 95

P

Pancetta Chicken, 66

Peanuts/peanut butter. *See* Nuts and seeds

Pears
  Thai Steak & Pear Salad, *90–91*
  Zippy Pear Veggie Rolls, 37

Peppers
  about: roasting, 95
  Chipotle Orange Chicken, *72–73*
  Garden-Vegetable Omelet Filling, 25
  Grilled Pork Tenderloin & Peppers, *100–101*
  Red Pepper & Goat Cheese Omelet Filling, 25
  Red Pepper-Basil Veggie Rolls, 37

Peppers (continued)
  Roasted Shrimp & Poblano
    Salad, 116–117
  Smoky Chipotle Deviled
    Eggs, 45
  Spanish Chicken & Peppers,
    76–77
  Sweet Pepper Sauce, 85
  Western Omelet Filling, 25
Percents (ratios) of
  macronutrients, 9
Pesto, 139
Pesto-Bacon Deviled Eggs, 44
Physical activity, 11
Pickled and fermented foods,
  friendly to diet, 12
"Popcorn," cauliflower, 39
Pork. See also Sausage
  about: chopping bacon easily,
    29
  Bacon & Eggs Over
    Asparagus, 103
  Bacon Cheddar Bombs, 48
  Cod, Cabbage & Bacon in
    Parchment, 121
  Crustless Quiche Lorraine,
    28–29
  Glazed Bacon-Wrapped
    Turkey Breast, 70–71
  Grilled Pork Tenderloin &
    Peppers, 100–101
  Grilled Pork Tenderloin
    with Grainy Mustard
    Vinaigrette, 104–105
  Grilled Pork with Charred
    Harissa Broccoli, 98
  Ham & Cheese Deviled
    Eggs, 44
  Nutty Green Beans &
    Asparagus with Bacon,
    132–133
  Pancetta Chicken, 66
  Pesto-Bacon Deviled Eggs, 44
  Pork Chops with Rosemary-
    Truffle Sauce, 106–107
  Spanish Pork Pinchos
    Morunos, 102
  Spinach & Prosciutto Frittata
    Muffins, 22–23
Poultry, 53–79
  about: overview of recipes, 53;
    searing and glazing, 57
  Buffalo Chicken Cobb Salad,
    136–137
  Chicken Caprese, 75
  Chicken Souvlaki Skewers, 63
  Chicken with Creamy
    Spinach & Artichokes, 62
  Chipotle Orange Chicken,
    72–73
  Cilantro-Lime Chicken, 74
  Crispy Chicken with White
    Wine Pan Sauce, 52, 57
  Fiery Kung Pao Chicken,
    68–69
  Glazed Bacon-Wrapped
    Turkey Breast, 70–71

Lemony Herb Roast Chicken,
  64–65
Lighter Chicken Cacciatore,
  60–61
Moroccan Chicken with
  Preserved Lemons &
  Olives, 78–79
Mushroom Chicken Skillet
  with Herbed Cream Sauce,
  58–59
Nigerian Peanutty Suya
  Skewers, 56
Pancetta Chicken, 66
Roasted Baby Vine Tomato
  Grilled Chicken, 54–55
Spanish Chicken & Peppers,
  76–77
Spicy Jerk Drumsticks, 67
Protein, ratios for keto diet, 9

Ranch Dressing, 139
Raspberries, in Berry Blast
  Smoothie, 30
Ratios of macronutrients
  (macros), 9
Reactions from keto diet, 8–9
Red peppers. See Peppers
Roasted Baby Vine Tomato
  Grilled Chicken, 54–55
Roasted Salmon with Tomatoes
  & Green Beans, 118–119
Roasted Shrimp & Poblano
  Salad, 116–117
Roasting vegetables (by veggie
  type), 95
Rosemary-Truffle Sauce, 107
S
Salads
  about: overview of vegetable
    and salad recipes, 125
  Buffalo Chicken Cobb Salad,
    136–137
  Feta-Dill Greek Caesar,
    126–127
  Grape Tomato, Olive & Feta
    Salad, 32, 35
  Grilled Southwest Steak
    Salad, 82
  Lemony Brussels Sprout
    Salad, 130–131
  Pesto, 139
  Ranch Dressing, 139
  Roasted Shrimp & Poblano
    Salad, 116–117
  Soy-Braised Beef & Tomato-
    Mint Salad, 86–87
  Tapas Salad, 128
  Thai Steak & Pear Salad,
    90–91
  Warm Goat Cheese Salad, 138
  Wilted Kale Salad, 128
Salmon. See Fish
Salsa-Avocado Omelet Filling,
  24
Sauces
  about: making best-ever pan
    sauce, 94

Grainy Mustard Vinaigrette,
  105
Herbed Cream Sauce, 59
Ranch Dressing, 139
Rosemary-Truffle Sauce, 107
Sweet Pepper Sauce, 85
White Wine Pan Sauce, 57
Sausage
  Sausage-Stuffed Zucchini
    Boats, 108–109
  Smoky Manchego Bombs, 47
  Tapas Salad, 128
  Tuscan Sausage & Kale
    Frittata, 14, 19
Sautéed Spinach with Garlic, 129
Savory Dill Cheese Balls, 43
Savory Herb Ricotta, 41
Scale, food, 13
Scrambled Eggs with Cream
  Cheese, 18
Seafood. See Fish
Seared Steak with Blistered
  Tomatoes, 94
Searing and glazing meat/
  poultry, 57
Sesame Smoked Salmon Bombs,
  46
Skewers
  Chicken Souvlaki Skewers, 63
  Lebanese Kafta Kebabs, 110
  Nigerian Peanutty Suya
    Skewers, 56
  Spanish Pork Pinchos
    Morunos, 102
  Tomato & Mozzarella Bites,
    34–35
Smoky Chipotle Deviled Eggs,
  45
Smoky Manchego Bombs, 47
Smoothies, 30, 31
Soy-Braised Beef & Tomato-Mint
  Salad, 86–87
Spanish Chicken & Peppers,
  76–77
Spanish Pork Pinchos Morunos,
  102
Spiced Citrus Ricotta, 41
Spices and herbs, 12
Spicy Jerk Drumsticks, 67
Spicy Soy-Glazed Salmon,
  122–123
Spinach
  Chicken with Creamy
    Spinach & Artichokes, 62
  Green Light Juice, 31
  Sautéed Spinach with Garlic,
    129
  Spinach & Prosciutto Frittata
    Muffins, 22–23
Spiralizer, 13
Squash
  about: roasting zucchini, 95;
    thinly slicing summer
    squash, 21

Garden-Vegetable Omelet
  Filling, 25
Sausage-Stuffed Zucchini
  Boats, 108–109
Summer Squash Frittata,
  20–21
Veggie Rolls (with variations),
  37
Starting keto diet, 9
Summer Squash Frittata, 20–21
Sweet & Spicy Cheese Balls, 43
Sweeteners, 12
T
Tapas Salad, 128
Testing for ketosis, 11
Thai Steak & Pear Salad, 90–91
Tomatoes
  Chicken Caprese, 75
  Grilled Plumb Tomatoes, 83
  Roasted Baby Vine Tomato
    Grilled Chicken, 54–55
  Roasted Salmon with
    Tomatoes & Green Beans,
    118–119
  salads with. See Salads
  Seared Steak with Blistered
    Tomatoes, 94
  Tomato & Mozzarella Bites,
    34–35
Truffle Cauliflower "Popcorn," 39
Turkey breast, glazed bacon-
  wrapped, 70–71
Turnips, roasting, 95
Tuscan Sausage & Kale Frittata,
  14, 19
Two-Step Slow-Cooked Brisket,
  88–89
V
Vegetables. See also specific
  vegetables
  about: friendly to diet, 12;
    overview of salad and
    vegetable recipes, 125;
    roasting instructions by
    type, 95
  Garden-Vegetable Omelet
    Filling, 25
  Veggie Rolls (with variations),
    37
W
Warm Goat Cheese Salad, 138
Water, drinking, 9–11
Weight loss, keto diet for, 7, 8,
  9, 11, 13
Western Omelet Filling, 25
Whole foods to include in diet,
  12–13
Wild-Mushroom Beef Brisket,
  80, 84
Wilted Kale Salad, 128
Z
Zippy Pear Veggie Rolls, 37
Zucchini. See Squash

Metric Conversion Charts

The recipes that appear in this cookbook use the standard United States method for measuring liquid and dry or solid ingredients (teaspoons, tablespoons, and cups). The information in these charts is provided to help cooks outside the US successfully use these recipes. All equivalents are approximate.

METRIC EQUIVALENTS FOR DIFFERENT TYPES OF INGREDIENTS

STANDARD CUP	FINE POWDER (e.g., flour)	GRAIN (e.g., rice)	GRANULAR (e.g., sugar)	LIQUID SOLIDS (e.g., butter)	LIQUID (e.g., milk)
¾	105 g	113 g	143 g	150 g	180 ml
⅔	93 g	100 g	125 g	133 g	160 ml
½	70 g	75 g	95 g	100 g	120 ml
⅓	47 g	50 g	63 g	67 g	80 ml
¼	35 g	38 g	48 g	50 g	60 ml
⅛	18 g	19 g	24 g	25 g	30 ml

¼ tsp	=						1 ml
½ tsp	=						2 ml
1 tsp	=						5 ml
3 tsp	=	1 tbsp	=		½ fl oz	=	15 ml
		2 tbsp	=	⅛ cup	1 fl oz	=	30 ml
		4 tbsp	=	¼ cup	2 fl oz	=	60 ml
		5⅓ tbsp	=	⅓ cup	3 fl oz	=	80 ml
		8 tbsp	=	½ cup	4 fl oz	=	120 ml
		10⅔ tbsp	=	⅔ cup	5 fl oz	=	160 ml
		12 tbsp	=	¾ cup	6 fl oz	=	180 ml
		16 tbsp	=	1 cup	8 fl oz	=	240 ml
		1 pt	=	2 cups	16 fl oz	=	480 ml
		1 qt	=	4 cups	32 fl oz	=	960 ml
					33 fl oz	=	1000 ml = 1 L

USEFUL EQUIVALENTS FOR DRY INGREDIENTS BY WEIGHT

(To convert ounces to grams, multiply the number of ounces by 30.)

1 oz	=	¹⁄₁₆ lb	=	30 g
2 oz	=	¼ lb	=	120 g
4 oz	=	½ lb	=	240 g
8 oz	=	¾ lb	=	360 g
16 oz	=	1 lb	=	480 g

USEFUL EQUIVALENTS LENGTH

(To convert inches to centimeters, multiply the number of inches by 2.5.)

1 in	=			2.5 cm		
6 in	=	½ ft	=	15 cm		
12 in	=	1 ft	=	30 cm		
36 in	=	3 ft	=	1 yd	=	90 cm
40 in	=			100 cm	=	1 m

USEFUL EQUIVALENTS FOR COOKING/OVEN TEMPERATURES

	Fahrenheit	Celsius	Gas Mark
Freeze Water	32°F	0°C	
Room Temperature	68°F	20°C	
Boil Water	212°F	100°C	
Bake	325°F	160°C	3
	350°F	180°C	4
	375°F	190°C	5
	400°F	200°C	6
	425°F	220°C	7
	450°F	230°C	8
Broil			Grill

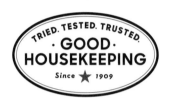

TESTED 'TIL PERFECT

Each and every recipe is developed in the Good Housekeeping Test Kitchen, where our team of culinary geniuses create, test, and continue to test recipes until they're perfect. (Even if we make the same dish ten times!)